For a first class nephew, To ~~~
with love
Stewart Wolf

Educating
DOCTORS

Stewart Wolf

Crisis in Medical Education, Research & Practice

Educating
DOCTORS

TRANSACTION PUBLISHERS
New Brunswick (U.S.A.) and London (U.K.)

Library of Congress Catalog Number: 96-29359
ISBN: 1-56000-301-4
Printed in the United States of America

Library of Congress Cataloging-in-Publication Data

Wolf, Stewart, 1914–
    Educating doctors : crisis in medical education, research, and practice / Stewart Wolf.
        p. cm.
    Includes bibliographical references and index.
    ISBN 1-56000-301-4 (alk. paper)
    1. Social medicine—United States. 2. Medicine—Philosophy. 3. Medical education—United States.   4. Medicine—Research—United States. 5. Holistic medicine. I. Title.
    [DNLM: 1. Education, Medical—United States. 2. Research—United States. 3. Delivery of Health Care. 4. Social Medicine. W 18
W855e 1996]
RA418.3.U6W65 1996
362.1'0973—dc20
DNLM/DLC
for Library of Congress   96-29359
                                                                                    CIP

Contents

List of Tables

List of Figures

Preface

This book is offered as a critique of the medical establishment and the way those concerned with its various responsibilities discharge them. I have tried to put in historical perspective and in relation to social changes the challenges and the methods devised for meeting medicine's responsibilities to society. Parts of the essays that follow have been compiled from editorials and commentaries published by the author in various books and medical journals over the past fifty years. I begin with how candidates for a career in medicine are selected, continuing with a commentary on currently designed teaching and learning, the qualities required in a physician and in a medical scientist, and the nature and the challenges of disease and what to do about them. Finally, I have tried to provide a useful way of thinking about human biology, to better understand why we are sick or well and what we have to contend with to stay well. Throughout, I have emphasized the role of the brain in controlling behavior of all sorts, general and visceral. The content of the book is biased by a heavy emphasis on the regulatory power of the nervous system as it perceives and evaluates life experiences and influences learning, behavior, and susceptibility to disease. The goal of the book is not to supply a recipe for the achievement of better health, but to encourage learning toward a better understanding of ourselves, of our patients, and of the paths toward health.

A smart chimpanzee can learn a variety of skills and a parrot can learn to remember and repeat information but neither is capable of advancing our knowledge; neither are they capable of wise judgements. It is the power to discriminate and the ability to evaluate evidence that sets man apart from the apes. So does the power of imagination and the capacity for vision. Creative imagination and originality of thought are dangerous attributes, however. They upset people, especially professional supervisors and managers. They often provoke a kind of retaliation which, at times, has even led to the innovator's being put to death. Very few important intellectual advances have failed to arouse suspicion, hostility, or disapproval. Happily, there have been those who have placed the exercise of unfettered originality of thought and action above the need for approval. Those forward-looking individuals have brought us, among other social benefits, high quality medical education, research, and practice. The continuous challenge is to maintain quality and to encourage the exercise of creative imagination and the freedom to inquire. Freedom is such a simple word that, having uttered it, we may not realize how much has been said. By surrendering our freedom to social dogmas of all sorts we renounce leadership for management.

Within the space of a hundred years the average man in America, once largely self-reliant and responsible for his own welfare and that of his family, and to some extent, his community, has progressively and ineluctably become managed by society. In fact, our having yielded to the social power of management may have contributed to the loss of a sense of individual responsibility in our culture today.

At a time when medical care for the people of the U.S. is undergoing a wrenching change due mainly to vast and costly technological progress, the doctors have had to cede much of their initiative and responsibility to third parties. As a consequence medicine has become a commercial enterprise. Doctors are being hired in increasing numbers by hospitals, insurance companies, and entrepreneurs. Patients must affiliate themselves with one of these organizations in order to have access to their doctors. The straitened situation in which patients, physicians and hospitals find themselves is appropriately called managed care. The solo practitioner, accessible to any patient in need of care, is fast disappearing.

A heavy financial burden has fallen on profession and public alike. Perhaps the most radical split from tradition is evident in the commercial advertising by doctors, hospitals, and even the most distinguished American universities. The payment for this costly enterprise comes from the patients' insurance premiums. The profits go to the managers.

As inappropriate to the mission of medicine as these developments are, they are less destructive than is the impersonal nature of medical practice that they encourage. In the hurly-burly of today's techno-medicine, many physicians are too busy to spend time in dialogue with their patients. As a consequence, social and emotional circumstances that have been thoroughly documented to powerfully affect physiology and susceptibility to disease are overlooked. Diagnostic tests and procedures are replacing meticulous attention to the characteristics and needs of the unique individual. The patient's message is not heard. Medical practice in a cardiac clinic, for example, is beginning to approach the triage of the battlefield with its hurried transfer of patients to catheterization or to insensitive technological diagnostic procedures.

Many modern physicians will dispute this judgment and maintain that patients still enjoy a close trusting and comfortable relationship with their physician. That is certainly still true, but it is also true that HMOs prescribe the number of patients a physician must see each day, thereby forcing a uniform limitation of time the physician can spend with each patient. Cardiac surgeons are required by some hospitals to perform a stated number of heart bypass operations to maintain their staff membership.

Not only in medicine, but in other social institutions, management has become the touch stone to progress. Its power has been felt in the trade unions and in the government, starting with the post World War I income tax, in corporations, including those that today are managing doctors and hospitals, and now, more and more, in the educational institutions themselves. Finally, government offices and corporations have decreed managed care for the ambulatory sick.

Universities have been suffering an alarming proliferation of administrators that amounts to a costly scourge of management engulfing and suppressing what was once their raison d'etre, intellectual leadership. As we have thus far failed to learn from the collapse of the Soviet Union, leadership cannot exist under management. It must be the other way around. Managers are essential to efficient operation, but they must be led by the vision of those who understand the mission. The managers should have an important role to advise, organize, and expedite the work, but their authority should be subordinate to that of the educators whose job it is to inspire, encourage, and perfect the work of the faculty. Now, however, the education of medical students, research, and the practice of medicine are, because of the incursions of managers, hobbled and stultified by bureaucrats and bureaucratic thinking. Such regimentation of thought and action has caused physician and medical scientist alike to become less inspired and less in touch with their sense of dedication and responsibility to patients and to fresh and imaginative enquiry. In other words, management has curbed the individual's sense of responsibility and initiative.

Judge Roscoe Pound, dean of the Harvard Law School, in a lecture to the Massachusetts Medical Society (Pound, 1942) reminded his listeners, both teachers and researchers, that the goal of medicine is neither economic nor political, but simply "the practice of a learned art in pursuit of a public service."

This important public service, or what politicians refer to as "health care" has been undergoing scrutiny during the past few years, and especially during the current year. The inquiry has focused almost exclusively on cost and distribution rather than on quality or coverage. Not surprisingly, service entrepreneurs and insurance businesses have taken advantage of the potentially lucrative opportunity to buy or to hire doctors and to manage the "delivery of health care." It is therefore high time to set a new target with quality care for the patient at the bull's eye, high time to focus on excellence in medical education, research, and practice. To provide proper care for the patient in all the meanings of that word assumes an understanding of human biology and human vulnerability. The patient's message must be heard and heeded. The first concern is the education of the physician. The next is to encourage scientific inquiry with the ultimate aim of continually enhancing the quality of the practice of medicine.

My aim here is to reexamine the responsibilities, goals, and activities of medical teachers, researchers, and practitioners, and to encourage the reader to understand the problems facing medicine. I want also to emphasize the importance of good leaders and the limitations imposed when managers are in charge. I hope the reader will also look beyond the fetters of current social and scientific dogmas that restrict imagination and embrace a broader vision of the future potential of medical education, research, and practice. Dogmas have been built around new insights or discoveries ad seriatim since the earliest recorded documents about the human mind (soul) and body. Unfortunately, many dogmas have been extraordinarily tenacious, even in the face of well-documented and thorough refutation. Hence, those who have come forth with new theories and interpretations have usually met disbelief, ridicule or censure. Their work, therefore, becomes obscured by a dense overgrowth of often incorrect prevailing wisdom.

Chapter 1 states the necessary standards for the education of competent physicians, pointing out the need for the student to learn "the machinery of the body" and also the nature of the person within it. Our knowledge of body parts and how they work together, while far superior today than half a century ago, is still imperfect. Therefore the student of medicine must continue to study for a lifetime. Our knowledge of the nature of the person is also imperfect, but is growing slowly. Moreover, thanks to the burgeoning knowledge of the complex interactive neural network in the brain, studies of the person and the body are coming together. Chapter 2 addresses the relevance of this convergence to the practice of medicine.

As human behavior and especially human interrelationships are relevant to health and disease, medicine is a social science and must be practiced in relation to social needs, currents of change and the organization of society. Chapter 3 examines this relationship.

The primary and continuing source for medical education and for practice is research. Chapters 4 and 5 explore the vast scope of medical research. Chapter 6 reviews what we have learned about health and disease from centuries of study and experience. Here the emphasis is on biological adjustments that adapt the organism to a wide variety of perturbations during the process of living. Here again the reader encounters intercommunications and interactions between the brain "the organ of the person," the structures of the body, and the social environment.

The storehouse for knowledge, its conveyer and, perhaps in the future, its synthesizer—the library—is celebrated in chapter 7. Chapter 8 deals with the multitude of triumphs and pitfalls encountered during the process of treating a sick patient. Most failures are found to stem from insufficient knowledge of the patient, inadequate attention to a detailed history and physical examination, and from reliance on technology as a substitute for thinking, in general, failure to grasp the patients message.

Chapter 9 describes the physiological complexity of bodily systems in the process of their adaptation to various pathogenic forces, including "the slings and arrows of outrageous fortune." It argues that human biology cannot be understood by the study of compartments and explains how the integrated mechanisms that keep us alive and well are regulated in the brain.

Contending with Dogmas

According to the account of the medical historian Logan Clendening (Clendening, 1960) Galen had once treated Marcus Aurelius for a digestive upset and so impressed him that the emperor complimented Galen as "one physician who was not hide-bound by rules." Ironically Galen's thorough anatomical studies created one of the longest lasting dogmas in the history of medicine. For more than a millennium, knowledge of human anatomy was delayed because data obtained from dissections of animals made by Galen in the second century AD were believed to apply to man. Not until the late thirteenth century and early fourteenth century did Mondino Di Lucci, professor of anatomy at Bologna introduce the study of human anatomy. He also wrote a manual on dissection. Over a century later Leonardo da Vinci produced even more elegant data on human anatomy.

The first comprehensive and fully organized study of human anatomy was published by Andreas Vesalius from what he learned by dissecting the bodies of executed criminals. Realizing that the dissection of dead bodies yielded no information on the functions of the viscera, however, Vesalius undertook to dissect living animals, mainly dogs. Thus, not only did Vesalius thoroughly revise the anatomy of Galen but, as a vigorous opponent of dogma, he also attempted to destroy the tenacious myth of the bone of Luz, a part of the right big toe, from which, it was believed, man would eventually be regenerated.

The Neglect of Available Paths of Inquiry

Unfortunately, important opportunities may be neglected because medical scientists are all too prone to the influence of current fashions—"What is hot? What is not?" and "What is getting generous funding?" For example, there are two long neglected hormones in the human body that have only recently been discovered to enhance the immune system and to exert possible powerful protection against diabetes, atherosclerosis, cancer and perhaps Alzheimer's disease and aging. Both agents were well known twenty-five years ago. Moreover, their molecular structure had been discovered and mapped, and yet their function in the bodily economy was not seriously investigated until quite recently. Somehow both hormones had failed to arouse the interest of most medical scientists because of a general agreement or dogma, that neither hormone was of great physiological significance.

One of the hormones, melatonin, is produced in the pineal gland. It was originally thought to regulate skin pigmentation. It does so in frogs, but not in humans. During the past five years it has been discovered to be one of the body's principal scavengers of free hydroxyl radicals, major oxidants implicated etiologically in several diseases.

The other hormone, dehydroepiandrosterone, (DHEA) was long known to be secreted by the adrenal cortex, and its molecular structure was also known years ago but its functions were not thought to be of great moment. Only during the past five years have we learned that DHEA is the major secretion of the adrenal cortex, responsible for modulating or perhaps inhibiting the effects of cortisol. The effects of both hormones are described in chapter 6.

The need for fresh, independent thinking in efforts to solve problems and the need to maintain an attitude of inquiry rather than one of absorption will be emphasized throughout this book. There are myriad problems in medical education, research, and practice waiting to be solved. They must be dealt with rigorously, wisely, and soon by responsible people in the government, public, and professional sectors if we are to avoid collapse of the system.

Acknowledgements

I am indebted to the following publishers for permission to reproduce here parts of my text and illustrations from their books and journals. Charles C. Thomas, University of Oklahoma Press, *Current Medical Digest, Transactions of the American Clinical and Climatological Association, The Pharos, JAMA, Clinical Research, The American Journal of Medicine, Psychosomatics, Integrative Physiological and Behavioral Sciences, The Pavlovian Journal, Clinical Research Proceedings*. Also, Oxford University Press, Johns Hopkins University Press, Transaction Publishers, The American Heart Association, Paul B. Hoeber, Williams and Wilkins, The American Physiological Society, The American Society of Pharmacology, University of Washington Press, Lippincott, *The New England Journal of Medicine*, The American Psychosomatic Society, Little Brown, and Lea & Febiger.

I am also grateful to Barbara Griffin for long hours of editorial assistance and critique and to Joy Lowe for preparing the manuscript and patiently tolerating seemingly endless rewrites and changes and to Peggy Chavis for her valuable advice and careful editing suggestions.

Finally I want to thank Irving Louis Horowitz, the president, Mary Curtis, the publisher, Sandra Klein-Suriano, former journals editor, Donna Kronemeyer, journals editor of Transaction Publishers, Camille Muhlbach for help with the bibliography and Thomas Wolf with the illustrations.

1

Medical Education

"The direction in which education starts a man will determine his future life."

—Plato

The Selection of Candidates for Medical School

Before World War II, selection among applicants to medical school was usually the responsibility of a single faculty member who was appointed because of his skill at interviewing and his reputation for perspicacity and good judgment. Such admissions officers in most medical schools were seeking mainly young men and women "of good character" with a broad liberal education. The applicant's level of academic achievement was also an important criterion but by no means were those with the highest grade point averages automatically admitted. The ability to think and to question are qualities essential to physician and researcher alike, but they do not necessarily equate with a high grade point average. A proper candidate for medical school must be susceptible to intellectual stimulation, engagement, and inspiration. The rapid grasp of a prehensile mind and the superior memory of a retentive mind are qualities that lead to high grade point averages, but neither is sufficient for an adequate medical education if reflective, inquisitive, and analytical qualities are missing. The demands of medicine, either in practice or research, have a closer resemblance to detective work than to a craft. An admissions officer's assessment of the candidate's motivation and intellectual breadth was more highly rated than was where in the upper third of his or her class the applicant stood. Moreover, having taken science courses to the neglect of a liberal education was usually a handicap to the applicant.

1

Applications to medical schools increased sharply in association with post-World War II social changes that included financial support for those who had served in the military to complete or enhance their education. Together with the enhanced student body, there occurred a large increase in the headquarters staff of the medical schools with a consequent shift in criteria for selection of students toward more bureaucratic standards. The admissions officers were replaced by a "representative" admissions committee. Fearing criticism for unfair discrimination, the committees sought defensible "objective" criteria and seized on grade point averages and scores on the medical college aptitude test. They were clearly numerical, but hardly reliable assessments of an applicant's qualifications for a medical education. Letters of recommendation from teachers, especially those dealing with character qualities, were largely ignored. Instead there was usually an interview of some sort conducted by casually selected faculty members or by the admissions committee as a whole, few of whom could claim any insight into the applicant's quality as a person who could be trusted with vulnerable patients and their apprehensive families.

It is no news that committees rarely generate wisdom, and yet we continue to appoint committees to make difficult decisions. This politically correct quantitative substitute for a careful and cogent method for screening aspiring medical students has encouraged an unfortunate influx of students attracted by the opportunity to assure themselves a comfortable income and a high social standing. Such tendencies have already become evident among a much too large proportion of practicing physicians and surgeons in this country. Although fifty years ago most deans and members of admission committees favored candidates with a broad social perspective and education in humanities, in medical school today such a background does not afford the same level of priority that it once did. As a result, few medical students have more than a rudimentary acquaintance with the humanities. This deficiency was evident even in William Osler's day. He stated not long before his death in 1919: "By the time their college studies are completed these students have often forfeited the intellectual challenges and rewards that study in the humanities could have afforded" (Osler, 1920).

Educating the Medical Student

The education of a physician involves, to a large extent, the shaping of attitudes, sensitivities, and perceptions. Helping a student absorb an adequate sample of accumulated knowledge of human biology to date is a formidable, but straightforward task. For the future practitioner, however, much more is required effectively to engage a patient in dialogue, to perceive subtle cues to the diagnosis, and to achieve therapeutic goals. Ideally this task calls for a certain erudition and an attitude of humility, optimism, warmth, and patience. The future medical scientist must cultivate not only the above qualities but the ability to ask relevant questions of nature, a firm respect for evidence, and a sensitivity to bias. Few teachers in today's medical schools have time to communicate such attitudes, information, and skills to medical students. Sorely needed are inspiring teachers as role models who spend time with the students on and off hours, in a reflective environment as well as at times of medical crisis. Hands-on experience is needed to learn any profession. It is essential to clinical training and should also be part of the instruction in sciences basic to medicine.

Attentuated Relationships between Student and Teacher and Student and Patient

Unfortunately, medical students have become somewhat depersonalized by virtue of their sheer numbers.[1] The increased size of medical school classes has inevitably lessened the opportunity for a master-apprentice relationship between faculty and student and has caused the loss of an important ingredient of a good education, the personal bond between student and teacher. Older physicians can recall, as a rich source of learning, unplanned and even casual contacts with teachers and patients in the clinic or the laboratory. The current trend toward shortening the curriculum and, at the same time standardizing it with what is euphemistically called a core, minimizes the opportunity for such leisure learning, the learning from "hanging around."

From roughly 1960 to 1980 the federal government, using the method of the carrot and stick, encouraged medical schools to accept larger classes and urged communities to establish more medical schools. The stated purpose was to provide better care and better access to it for those previously denied medical care, mainly in the rural areas and inner cities. Paradoxically, the enlargement of student enrollment and the expansion and proliferation of medical schools has brought more administrators, more bureaucracy, more salaried faculty, and more distance between student and teacher. Along with other post-World War II developments, the expansion has caused medical students to be less consistently in personal contact with a role model teacher. It also has limited supervised hands-on experience and reduced the opportunity for student research, making the whole educational process more passive. It thus encourages vicarious learning in the face of what we all know: the vitality of the educated man stems from his ability to inquire on his own.

To learn how to care for patients, students need to be in direct contact with them for a length of time sufficient to understand each one and the nature of the disease in question.

The student's opportunity to share clinical responsibility without interruption over a reasonable period of time has, however, been all but eliminated by economic forces impinging on hospital care. The length of a patient's stay is no longer decided by the doctor's judgment of his or her needs, but by the budget-based rules of managed care corporations. What has been lost is not only the welfare of the patient but the experience of daily responsibility for an inpatient that can engender in interns and resident physicians a strong sense of commitment to meticulous attention to detail, wise decision making, and gentle care of the patients. Moreover, the personal attention involved in such simple routines as taking blood for testing and starting intravenous infusions may serve to strengthen the student's sense of obligation to the patient. These opportunities for personal service waned when later they began to be shared with nurses and technicians. Also, after World War II, for the first time, many of the students had married. Inevitably, their attention, at a critical time in their development as physicians, had to be divided between patients and family. By the 1970s resident physicians were no longer in residence. Therefore, both they and the students spent far less time in the hospital than had their predecessors.

Weakening of Education in Preclinical Sciences

Education in medical science is being slighted, owing in part to the enlargement of medical school classes and the increased cost of laboratory participation. Instead of learning by doing in anatomy and cell biology, biochemistry, physiology, microbiology, and pharmacology in the laboratory, and pathology in the autopsy room under the guidance of faculty scientists, students are consigned to classrooms where they listen to lectures and watch videotaped demonstrations. These communication media will later be used for their postgraduate education by the representatives of pharmaceutical companies.[2] Although videotapes may greatly help students who are learning a technique, in the basic education of a physician they cannot substitute for hands-on experience. Tosteson's "New Pathway" at Harvard resurrects many successful pre-World War II learning methods, including reduced emphasis on lectures. It says nothing, however, about returning medical students to the basic science laboratories where they might polish what he referred to as their important "attitudes of skepticism and doubt" (Tosteson, 1990).[3]

Learning About Patients as People, the Diseases and Disorders that Affect Them, and How to Alleviate Their Suffering

As specialties have constricted the focus of medical educators, intellectual leaders and clinical virtuosi have become *rara aves* on medical faculties. Once abundant, they are sorely needed today. Dr. William Parson, an old friend and bona fide clinical virtuoso, rummaging through his archives, came upon a picture of himself taken together with eleven of his colleagues. The scene was a gathering of chairmen of departments of medicine in schools around the country forty years ago. Like Parson, most of them were clinical virtuosi, leading educators. Parson was so struck by the contrast with present-day clinical teachers that he wrote the following in an essay on role models (Parson, 1995).

This old photo has made me think of the critical role the department chairman played in the education and development of the medical student. To be sure, class size has increased and administrative responsibilities have achieved priorities. The responsibilities of the chairman seem profoundly altered. And something rich has gone.

It is not difficult to list the deficiencies in the past patterns. Nonetheless, we did do some things of value. Our peer group followed our own teachers and made time to teach the fundamental disciplines, physical diagnosis, and history taking. What better way to emphasize priorities!

And then, because clinical experience and clinical skills were prerequisites for appointment, the professor made "live" ward rounds at the patients' bedsides (not over the charts in the conference room) with clinical clerks and house staff. These involved the professor in demonstrating sensitivity to the patient, eliciting key points in the development of the illness, illustrating the examination of the patient, analyzing the diagnostic features (before selecting laboratory studies!), and reviewing the management of the case.

Grand rounds were great events and well attended (without the inducement of free lunches and handouts from the pharmaceuticals). They were not delegated; they were the professor's show. The patient was present to highlight key points in the presentation and answer some questions.

The discussion was developed around the patient's problem and its management. These were memorable learning experiences and different from the current pattern of a "dry" presentation used as a justification for "another medical school lecture."

Nostalgia surely blunts the memory. It seems clear, however, that we faculty members knew more about more of the students then, and they certainly knew who the professor was and what the priorities were.

Role models almost seem politically incorrect today. In any event, there was a dynamic relationship with the student. We could be accepted or rejected, but not ignored.

The Clinical Residency

William Osler's signal contribution to medical education was the hospital residency by which, while learning by doing, young physicians could grow through graduated stages of clinical responsibility. In a thoughtful and well-documented essay, Alan Astrow traces the beginnings of such patient-centered clinical training to France before and during the Revolution (Astrow, 1990). Building on an idea proposed in 1778 by two prominent French physicians, Claude-François Duchanoy and Jean-Baptiste Junelin, Philippe Pinel, in 1793 proposed a pattern for clinical teaching that combined an emphasis on twenty-four-hour availability to patients, personalized, humane care, and research (Pinel, 1908). Pinel's design was institutionalized in 1802 during the Empire by Napoleon's minister of the interior, Jean Antoine Chaptal, and prescribed that a hospital-trained physician should have "the inquisitive attitude of an anthropologist as well as a zoologist" and should become "consoler of the suffering and the weak, indifferent to fame and wealth, subservient only to his conscience and patriotic duty" (Staum, 1980). Astrow believed that the need for precise observation of patients to further the science of medicine would require that the teaching physicians control the management of their hospitalization, an arrangement he viewed as having encroached on the independence and freedom of choice of the patients. He further speculated that, as physicians in charge focused more and more on the heuristic value of a patient's physical disturbances for teaching and research, they may have become less attentive to the needs of the individual, thereby gradually corrupting medical education to the point of "losing its soul." It would not be difficult to find hospitalized patients today who would quickly agree with Astrow's formulation, but whether erosion of the patients' freedom of choice or, alternatively, whether diffusion of responsibility in the care of patients has contributed most to corrupting medical education is not immediately evident.

For at least a century after the Revolution, members of the French medical establishment engaged in a dispute about whether the emphasis in medical education should be "practical" or "academic." In the United States, with the strong support of the American Medical Association, founded in 1847, the exponents of the practical held sway until the opening of the Johns Hopkins Medical School in 1893. The Hopkins gave a powerful boost to the scientific emphasis in medical education and viewed the hospital as a resource, not only for teaching the care of patients but also for advancing knowledge through careful study of what mechanisms were responsible for disabilities. William Osler described his residency program as providing "an education that begins with the patient, continues with the patient and ends...with the patient, using books and lectures as tools, as a means to an end" (Osler, 1903). Osler's method depended heavily on having a relatively small number of students in each class (Rothstein, 1987). "With a small class I have been satisfied with the results, "wrote Osler, "but the plan would be difficult to carry out with a large body of students."

I was exposed to the Oslerian approach to clinical teaching as a medical student at Johns Hopkins from 1934 to 1938. Although William Osler himself had left more than twenty years before to become Regius Professor of Medicine at Oxford, most of the still-active senior faculty in the Department of Medicine who had been taught by Osler and whom he had heavily influenced by his standards and his traditions were still there. Many of the existing faculty had visited or had worked in European clinics following their early medical training at Hopkins or elsewhere. These richly educated professors were willing and able to spend time with individual students since each class contained only about seventy students. Then the science of medicine was growing apace, and basic physiological and chemical mechanisms were emphasized in clinical teaching, as were civility and good communication with patients. Francis Peabody, who had studied under William Osler at Hopkins, in 1921 became the first director of the Thorndike Memorial Laboratory at Harvard affiliated with the fourth ward service at Boston City Hospital. That institution became the most distinguished research and teaching department in the United States. Peabody, clearly no enemy of science in medicine, championed the view that personal interest and an understanding of the patient are fundamental to good practice (Peabody, 1930).

A further effort to inculcate an attitude of inquiry into young physicians in training was pursued at the University of Oklahoma in line with the view of Harvard's Dr. Henry Christian—that if you let a young person work somewhat on his own, he will eventually come up with something. While emphasis was placed on clinical experience in bedside and ambulatory medicine with increasing responsibility year after year, the residents were encouraged to identify themselves from the very beginning with an individual interest. To assist in this aim we established, close to the ward on the main traffic arteries of the University hospital, five "project rooms" where the attitude of inquiry held sway. Each of these specialty conference room-laboratories was supervised by one of the sub-department heads. Under this system it was easy for the students and house officers to maintain a close colleague relationship with one of the faculty (Wolf, 1956).

In these project rooms there was appropriate equipment with which special studies on patients could be carried out and many questions answered. Consultation and guidance were available from the teacher-investigator who spent a part of each day in the project room and from the research fellows and residents permanently assigned to these services. Students and house officers often came in to chat and went out filled with enthusiasm for pursuing some question or clearing up a point at issue. The goal of the project room was to allow the residency experience to engage the aptitudes and serve the needs of the individual as well as to encourage his or her inclinations. The strategy worked well as is evident from the subsequent careers of those who took seriously their opportunities in the project rooms.

Foreshortening of the Clinical Residency

During and for a few years after World War II, an alternative to military service was established for especially promising residents in training in university hospitals. It appears that clinical education in medicine was slighted for some who have since risen to leadership positions in academic medicine. Called the Berry Plan, this arrangement allowed for the appointment of young physicians to the U.S. Public Health Service after they had completed only two or three years of hospital training. Many of them were assigned to the intramural laboratories of the NIH where their efforts were focused on a sharply restricted problem such as the purification of a single enzyme. Their clinical experience was often restricted to caring for a few selected patients in a narrow subspecialty in medicine. Such a narrow opportunity to study symptom-producing disturbances of physiological adaptative patterns in a single organ system restricts learning because the organ systems are interactive and their regulation is centrally integrated in the brain.

Many of those talented young people, whose clinical education had been truncated but intensified in a very restricted area, eventually joined the clinical faculties of medical schools. Many of them served as division heads or even department chairmen. Such doctors were poorly equipped to make teaching rounds on the general medicine services. Their limited clinical experience seemed to accentuate an already prevalent tendency among young physicians to "cover themselves" by asking for the consultation of specialists or for a battery of "scattergun" tests and procedures. Responsibility for the care of individual patients was thus diffused. It still is today as resident physicians in medicine are accepted for specialty training after a relatively brief exposure to the broad range of sick people.

Prior to World War II and before specialty boards took over the reins, clinical education was planned and managed by the clinical departments in medical schools. The ablest among medical residents were selected for the post of chief resident in their fifth year of house staff service. Having lived in the hospital throughout that period, they had become well seasoned and usually capable of the intellectual and interpersonal challenges of a medical practice or a junior academic post. After the American Board of Internal Medicine became fully established, it required only three years of hospital training for certification in internal medicine. This minimum training became the ceiling for most general internists who are practicing today. Not surprisingly, many of them lack the diagnostic maturity necessary to exploit the rich mine of clinical information available in a proper medical history. When the history is a skillfully managed exploratory dialogue with a patient it may yield crucial diagnostic information and give clues to where the subsequent physical examination should focus special attention. The narrowed education and experience of such young physicians deprived them of the richest elements of the art of medicine.

The Fine Art of Taking a History

"So productive of insight, so apparently simple, so truly complex: taking the history involves analysis and interpretation and requires the highest order of medical skill. Of all the technical aids that increase the doctor's power of observation, none comes even close in value to the skillful use of spoken words of the patient. Throughout all of medicine, use of words is still the main diagnostic technique."

—Brian Bird (1955)

Clearly, the most powerful diagnostic tool is the medical history, the dialogue with the patient. Periodically over the past several years, I have asked successful consultants what helped them most when they were able to make a diagnosis that had been missed by the referring physician. Nearly always the crucial clue came, not from a laboratory test or questionnaire, but from something the patient said. Thus, the dialogue that contains the history taking process becomes the single most crucial aspect of the diagnosis. It should include a "noninvasive" summary of the patient's background, early experiences, aspirations, ambitions, and vulnerabilities. Such information, as it brings the patient into focus as a person, can greatly facilitate the shrewd and sensitive inquiry needed to elicit an informative account of the illness and it may point to the relevance of further inquiry and could even facilitate therapy.

A history taken from a twenty-four-year-old man is illustrative of the failure to heed a potentially significant lead in the dialogue. For the previous eight weeks the patient had been experiencing anorexia, nausea, and vomiting so severe that he had lost more than twenty pounds. His symptoms had begun on the day of his marriage. Further questioning elicited another concurrent problem: premature ejaculation. The examiner, a medical student, jumped to the conclusion that there was a disturbance in the patient's psychosexual development—perhaps ambivalence about his role as a man or even a homosexual tendency. Accordingly, he carefully reviewed the patient's early sexual experience, inquired extensively about his first meeting with his wife, their courtship, and their wedding night. The patient answered all questions in an earnest and frank manner, obviously trying to cooperate, but was unable to turn up anything pertinent. Fortunately, the interview had been recorded, and on replay the student picked up the clue he had missed while taking the family history. A portion of the exchange follows:

Q: You're married?

A: Yes, I was married June 24.

Q: Was your wife from Omaha?

A: No, she was from Fort Madison but we married in Omaha, hoping my mother would come. She only gets around in a wheelchair.

Q: Yes, you mentioned that she had an accident. You have no children then?

The history of the family was completed with the student having missed the significant lead: "hoping my mother would come." At the next visit, with more listening and fewer questions, the pertinent part of the story quickly unfolded. The patient's mother had been rendered paraplegic in an automobile accident that occurred while he was driving. He had been seriously injured as well but had recovered. His mother apparently adjusted to her disability remarkably well and gave no indication of resentment toward him. His father had died two years earlier.

An older brother and two older sisters were married, so the patient had continued to live at home. His mother ran the household and had a nurse and a maid to look after her personal needs. She had never shown any particular enthusiasm for any of the young women in whom he was interested, but she had been pleasant and cordial whenever he brought one of them to the house. When he finally became engaged, she seemed to accept the prospect of marriage but gave no special encouragement. He was uneasy and felt guilty about leaving her.

Her failure to appear at the wedding, especially arranged by the bride's parents to be conveniently accessible to his mother, was a severe blow to the patient. He had managed to repress most of his feelings, however, until during the second interview the student raised the question about his mother's failure to attend the wedding. Then, as the realization struck him, he wept a bit and talked a great deal. The student listened and reassured the patient that his mother was naturally frightened of, and perhaps angry at, losing him but that she would probably accept this event with equanimity as she had accepted other difficult situations in the past.

The student's speculations about the mother ultimately proved to be true. The patient's symptoms improved rapidly. They had reflected an alarming gastrointestinal disturbance that could not have been explained by any amount of laboratory testing, x-ray, or endoscopy, but they were illuminated by—and ultimately yielded to—a skillfully conducted interview. Such important diagnostic information may emerge, not only from direct responses to questions, but also from a host of verbal and nonverbal clues that somewhat resemble the value of presystolic rumbles heard during auscultation of the heart.

The presystolic crescendo rumble heard through the stethoscope is a highly reliable, almost conclusive sign of mitral stenosis. That remarkably dependable information about the condition of the mitral valves is nevertheless indirect. One cannot see or feel the mitral leaflets. Moreover, it requires a practiced ear to detect and identify a presystolic rumble. Likewise, there are comparable and equally reliable "presystolic rumbles" detectable by the practiced ear in listening to the patient. They include unconscious revelations of context, slips of the tongue, contradictions, and other subtle clues from the way things are said or left unsaid and from replies that are evasive, defensive, or irrelevant. To detect such clues the physician must cultivate patience and understanding and sharpen all senses to be alert for what is hidden.

Thus, communication with patients is the very essence of the doctor's job. Lectures and written examinations do very little to promote such skills. Moreover, once in practice, the physician learns that, except to psychiatrists, third-party payers provide no adequate compensation for verbal communication with patients. Thus, with no financial incentive for a skillful and penetrating interview, the physician may assign history taking to a surrogate and adopt the widely prevalent practice of placing primary reliance for diagnosis on laboratory tests and special procedures. He thereby not only fails to gather potentially important, or even crucial, clinical data but misses the satisfaction of personal involvement in a successful effort to get to the bottom of a patient's illness.

Unfortunately, some physicians have come to believe that computer-aided histories and questionnaires have, not only better memory and reproducibility but better discrimination than does the interview. They are overlooking the unique feature of the brain, the human computer that can catch subtle cues and can change pace or direction to pursue a pertinent lead toward the solution of the individual patient's problem. Such clues, gathered from the history and from the physical examination as well, may be altogether inaccessible to chemical screening tests, scans, or other technical procedures. Sad to say, an impersonal diagnostic effort has a certain appeal to young doctors in training. It saves the student's time and protects him from the intellectual challenge to understand their patient and his or her medical problem. Not only in America, but in Europe as well, students are welcoming the opportunity to diminish or pass over the indispensible diagnostic dialogue. A recently received French periodical, *Le Quotidien du Medicin*, for February 27, 19967 states: "examining the patient no longer interests medical students. The senior physicians who serve as models for the the students...after assessing the problem by a few questions to the patient, turn at once to the ordering of tests."

Beyond its importance in diagnosis, effective communication with patients through history taking may enhance the quality of the patient-physician relationship. In direct contact with the patient, the student can learn to keep his intellectual motor running, so to speak, considering likely diagnoses from the moment of his first greeting the patient. Diagnostic impressions can then undergo progressive modifications as conjectures that do not fit the accumulating data are discarded. The surviving probabilities should then be tested in the laboratory or by a suitable diagnostic procedure. Like Sherlock Holmes, the good diagnostician looks for features in a case that do not fit what may seem to be a plausible diagnosis. Less astute physicians, like Conan Doyle's Sergeant Lestrade, failing to heed a crucial clue, miss the correct diagnosis by simply compiling the evidence and settling on a diagnosis that seemed to be in keeping with the preponderance of the data. The right answer is reached more often by the relentless pursuit of a highly reliable bit of evidence that, as Sherlock Holmes taught us, does not fit the initial assumption.

Teaching the Art of Medicine

What is the attending physician expected to contribute to the educational process during ward rounds? His proper job is to teach the art of medicine, to help students and residents enhance their capabilities for clinical analysis and synthesis, to sharpen their sensitivity to clues and to the individual needs of their patients. At the bedside he can convey to the students his skill and experience in relating to patients and eliciting and evaluating clinical data.

Art is an elusive concept, whether reflecting the work of a Rembrandt, a Calder, or a musical virtuoso such as Itzhak Perlman, or, in medicine, an Osler. The physician's art is often seen in contrast to his science, being recognizable in the elicitation of placebo responses or in a bedside manner that encourages optimism and engenders in patients a sense of well being. The art of medicine includes these but goes well beyond them, beyond diplomacy, kindness, and caring to include the skill with which a physician elicits and evaluates evidence, charts a course for the management of his patient's illness, and the way he or she inspires students.

Such clinical virtuosi will be recognized on ward rounds by their ability to synthesize, to pick up and put together clues that might elude a less skillful colleague, and by their ability to engender a comfortable and secure atmosphere in which effective and understanding communication with patients and their families can take place. Such broadly educated teachers once flourished on medical school faculties but nowadays are less frequently encountered since the responsibility for the welfare of patients has become fragmented among specialists.

Unfortunately, ward rounds in teaching hospitals are taking place more and more in chart rooms or conference rooms in front of x-ray view boxes, and less and less at the bedside (Linfors & Neelon, 1980). Therefore, the teacher must accept what he is told. With only x-rays, scans, and laboratory tests available to him and without firsthand access to the data gathering process, the ability of the attending physician to teach the recognition of subtle clues available during communication with the patient and to share his analytical prowess with students and house officers is diminished.

Bureaucratic Restraints to Independent Thought and Learning

Progress in any field is dependent upon freedom of thought, not upon the possession of passports stamped by an approving authority. As pointed out earlier, education differs from training in that it is fecund, productive. It is also, in a sense, cumulative. There have always been attempts by authorities to restrict people's minds. Today the medical teacher is hemmed in on both sides by powerful, approving (and disapproving) forces. To survive in research the investigator must satisfy the study sections of the NIH. To work with students and house officers he or she must earn the approval of the various visiting teams of the American

Medical Association and specialty boards. But there is danger in undue emphasis on peer approval. Dr. Alan Gregg, in referring to the Specialty Board of Internal Medicine, once told a gathering of the American College of Physicians: "the tradition of examinations in this country is not to find out what a candidate knows, but whether he knows what his examiners know.... Every tendency in our profession, especially every trend that seeks to strengthen its position by means of standardization, obligatory uniformity and unvarying acceptance deserves to be challenged as a threat to variety and survival" (Gregg, 1949).

Freedom of thought in exploration of new territories requires courage. Several years ago, in a commencement address at the University of Colorado, I quoted from a movie scenario by Dylan Thomas (Thomas, 1945). The story is about Rock, a professor of anatomy in a medical school during the Middle Ages. He had lost his job because of laws passed by the politicians and the clerics who had made it close to impossible to obtain human bodies to dissect. Thus, thinking that their doctors could learn all they needed by poring over the books of Galen and perpetuating the errors and misinformation contained therein, they effectively prohibited the true study of human anatomy. Rock, the professor of anatomy, like most of his colleagues, was working with human bodies exhumed illegally by ghouls who earned their living by grave robbing. Unfortunately, one of the men working for Rock became overzealous and began to provide bodies that had skipped the formality of natural death and burial. This man was caught killing off the denizens of skid row and selling them to Rock. Of course, it was Rock, who had known nothing of these crimes, who suffered for them when they were found out and it was Rock who lost his job at the university. The movie scenario picks him up as he is giving his last lecture to his class. Let me quote from Dylan Thomas:

As the camera moves over the heads of the class toward the front of the lecture hall, the figure of Rock fills the screen and he is saying: 'To think, then, is to enter into perilous country, colder of welcome than the polar wastes, darker than a Scottish Sunday, where the hand of the unthinker is always raised against you, where the wild animals, who go by such names as Envy, Hypocrisy, and Tradition, are notoriously carnivorous, and where the parasites rule.

To think is dangerous. The majority of men have found it easier to writhe their way into the parasitical bureaucracy, or to droop into the slack ranks of the ruled. I beg you all to devote your lives to danger; I pledge you to adventure; I command you to experiment. Remember the practice of Anatomy is absolutely vital to the progress of medicine. Remember, that the progress of medicine is vital to the progress of mankind. And mankind is worth fighting for: killing and lying and dying for. Forget what you like. Forget all I have ever told you. But remember that.

The wild animals that threaten today's medical school graduates go by such names as Information Overload, Prescribed Learning, and Approving Authority. Some of them lurk among the drastic changes in medical school curricula that prescribe an "indispensable" core of information and knowledge, command of which is to be tested "objectively." Moreover, important intangible qualities of students, not susceptible to objective assessment, such as reliability, honesty, dedication, perspicacity, understanding, and interest in patients are often lost sight of.

The faculties of some schools have now become aware that their overstructuring of the curriculum has not accelerated the pace or contributed to the quality of learning. In an earlier day, the period from 1880 to 1912, American medical education advanced with almost explosive speed. It was a time when ambitious young physicians applied themselves to what might be called open-ended learning without curricula or qualifying requirements. They learned from "hanging around" and from myriad, unplanned exposures to special people, ideas, and experience. At the turn of the century young American doctors, innocents abroad, visited and worked in the great laboratories and clinics of Europe, electing and digesting their experiences in their own way. Returning home, they brought forth on this continent a new and vital form of medical education that in turn made America the "Mecca." These scholars, preparing to be teachers, understood that the proper function of the educator is procreation, not duplication. Intellectual conformity may confer a sense of belonging and of acceptance by one's fellows but often at the sacrifice of freshness and originality. Carried to an extreme, efforts to gain acceptance can result in a continuous intellectual minuet in which we bow to each other and walk around arm in arm according to a cadence that cannot be broken for risk of disapproval.

Education properly encourages both high standards and diversity in learning, in inquiry, and in interpretation. Lewis Moorman, an outstanding medical scholar and one-time dean of the University of Oklahoma School of Medicine, compared the modern scholar to a squirrel: "He should be free to garner the best from the topmost boughs of the boundless forest. Committed to the annulling tread of conformity within the confines of a miserable cage, however, he cracks only the nuts supplied by his keeper" (Moorman, 1954). Emerson, in these words, saw the business of cracking only nuts supplied by a keeper: "Men grind and grind in the mill of a truism, and nothing comes out but what was put in. But the moment they desert the tradition for a spontaneous thought, then poetry, wit, hope, virtue, learning, anecdote, all flock to their aid" (Emerson, 1838). Unfortunately, those with creative imagination are not always equally endowed with courage. Too many of us walk voluntarily into the cage of conformity. It takes a hardy soul to withstand the pressure of disapproval and continue running on the topmost bough.

Barriers We Create

Few of us approach our potential for education, for personal cultivation. Those who have done so have usually been inspired by another individual or by a rich personal experience. One reason for the failure of some to approach their potential may be traced to having encountered unnecessary walls built by ourselves.

America's beloved poet Robert Frost was questioning an old tradition that held that "good fences make good neighbors" (Frost, 1950). "Why do they make good neighbors?" asked Frost.

It is a good question. What are we fencing in or out? Walls and fences are like categories and points of view that have crystallized. They come along naturally in the course of man's utilization of the riches of nature, but eventually they seem to develop an importance and significance of their own. We erect some walls for a variety of questionable purposes, such as the exclusion of individuals from membership in learned societies. Most such societies were organized on the basis of the human impulse for kindred minds to gather in groups to exchange ideas. Later came the search for new members of the society. Then, after the society has gained glory and prestige, there comes the stage of exclusion to serve the human need for a sense of being elite.

Apart from walls to serve human vanity are the walls of tradition that set a limit on man's capacity to approach the truth. The synthesis of urea from ammonia by Friedrich Wöhler (1800–1882) in 1828 broke through what had seemed an impenetrable wall of tradition. At that time a longstanding dogma held that such chemicals were components of human organisms and could never be made by man. That is, while inorganic compounds could be synthesized, organic compounds could not, because they contained a vital ingredient beyond man's reach.

Even Pasteur, a free mind in medicine, undertook some wall-building when he spoke to the French Academy at the time of his election to that body that had earlier scorned him. As he entered the Academy's high walls of prestige and acceptance, he said that scientific method is not applicable to problems involving emotions. Within a very few years of this pronouncement Pavlov and later Walter Cannon were chipping away at Pasteur's wall that would have limited man's capacity to approach the truth. As Robert Frost put it, "Something there is that doesn't love a wall, that wants it down."

Aesthetics and Humanities as Vitamins in Medical Education

Albert Jonsen has called attention to a lecture given by William Osler not long before his death in 1919. In it he likened the effect of the humanities on medical progress to hormones, a word derived from the Greek meaning to excite or stimulate (Jonsen, 1989; Osler, 1920). His implication was that a liberal education engenders breadth of intellectual development and personal commitment to human service.

There is also a striking parallel between the function of vitamins in the bodily economy and that of aesthetics and humanities in human development. Vitamins provide no calories and therefore no fuel for the body but are, nevertheless, essential to health. A person deprived of vitamins can gain weight, even become obese, but not be healthy. One deprived of aesthetic experience can become rich, even be admired and powerful, but not be fulfilled.

Steven Muller, former president of Johns Hopkins University, has suggested that exposure to aesthetics and humanities contributes to the development of values that not only guide behavior but provide significance and enrichment to one's activities and, to a large extent, define the qualities of a person (Muller, 1980). In his view, "the biggest failing in higher education today is that we fall short in exposing students to values."

Values may be defined as what we hold dear, believe in, live by, or risk our lives for. Our values derive from human experience in communicating with others and from learning. Learning values must certainly begin with early life experiences in the home and the church, in the schools, in associations with others, and in coping with life situations. To a large extent, however, values derive from connections with the past. Before the days of recorded history, poetry, and literature, value systems were passed along from generation to generation in stories, songs, dances, rituals of various sorts, and in such artistic works as painting and pottery design. Thereby were communicated not only appreciation of history, of forebears, of nature, and of human bonds but codes of behavior as well. Today, with historical, aesthetic, and ethical contributions widely available in print, there is less transmission of cultural traditions from generation to generation within the tribe and the family and less of a feel for history and tradition. According to Muller, many of today's college students are interested only in courses useful and relevant to a career, thereby incurring the risk of "our universities producing highly skilled barbarians" (Muller, 1980).

Perhaps the intellectual avitaminosis among college students is attributable in part to the fact that most pre-professional courses require only that the student learn a specified body of knowledge. Courses in the arts and humanities, on the other hand, require in addition that the student contribute some of his own thinking. The professors are not expecting right answers from the students but thoughtful responses, evaluations, and judgments. The educational experience in the humanities is, therefore, communicative rather than primarily acquisitive. By contributing something of himself or herself to the process, the student awakens perceptions and cultivates a sense of values and an ability to appreciate. The job of the teacher is presumably to enhance this ability. If universities are falling short in exposing students to courses that contribute to the development of values, what are the implications for medical schools?

Medical school catalogues often contain statements urging emphasis on liberal arts in premedical education. Moreover, admissions committees are often heard to express concern over the nature of the courses taken or of the intellectual aspirations of applicants to medical school. Nevertheless, these committees persist in using grade point averages as their primary criterion, continuing to favor applicants who have pursued Muller's "utilitarian route." These committees have thereby "shaped" the curriculum choices of college students toward those subjects where academic achievement can be measured on the basis of right and wrong answers. Courses in aesthetics and humanities are still avoided by the aspirant to medical school, because, as the student's performance is evaluated in terms of nonquantifiable insights, interpretations, and judgments, there is little assurance that the students can attain high grades by learning the right answers. Once a student is admitted to medical school, he or she faces further emphasis on the utilitarian. There is less chance for wonder, contemplation. Independent thought may be buried in the struggle to acquire information and have it ready for the next quiz. Thus, the need to develop attitudes toward serving people and the sensitivity to serve effectively may escape the student altogether.

Fortunately, some medical schools have recognized that, as vitamins contribute to the metabolic processes that build and maintain the integrity of tissues, so aesthetic experience contributes to educational growth and personal integrity. One such school is the University of Cincinnati, where Maurice Levine, former chairman of psychiatry, took a resolute antibarbarian stand. He invited, as regular participants in his department's educational program, poets, writers, historians, and philosophers. A former member of the Cincinnati family, W.B. Bean established an institute of medical humanities at the University of Texas Medical Branch in Galveston in 1972, and later Carlton Chapman did so at Albert Einstein College of Medicine in New York City. Other universities have finally made similar moves. Pennsylvania State University's College of Medicine was the first to initiate a department of humanities with courses in the curriculum. The importance of teaching literature in medical schools was recently underscored by Rita Charon and a group of collaborators from seven medical schools scattered across the country. In each of those institutions literature is part of the curriculum. They claim an important practical value of literature in medical education. Taking a strong position against the late nineteenth-century proposal of Thomas Huxley that natural sciences replace humane letters in general education, these authors document their case with outcome studies of the effects of their literature courses on medical students and physicians (Charon et al., 1995).

As encouraging as these developments seem, they are a late-course correction. Arts and humanities should be a part of education at all levels, including the lifelong continuing education of the physician. The artisan aspects of medicine must, of course, be mastered, but the physician must also be concerned with human values. Medicine, after all, is more than a science, more than an art or a profession; as it has to do with the fulfillment of a person, his health and well being, it is one of the humanities.

Notes

1. In 1960 there were 85 medical schools in the U.S. with a total of 30,288 students. By 1970 there were 41,487 students in 112 schools and by 1980, 65,189 students in 126 schools. In 1990, the number had decreased slightly to 65,163 students in 125 schools.

2. Most major pharmaceutical companies deploy an army of representatives called detail men. After receiving an intensive course of training concerning the chemical nature, physiological effects and clinical uses of each of the drugs to be promoted, the detail men seek personal interviews with physicians in practice and with faculty members in medical schools. After the interview the physicians are supplied with liberal quantities of samples for use on their patients. Since the information brought by the detail men is often new to the doctor, albeit biased, it has become a major aspect of postgraduate education for hosts of American physicians.

3. Tosteson's "New Pathway in General Medical Education" for the Harvard Medical School is more an emphasis than a plan. It calls for flexibility in medical education to enable students to cope with the rapidly accumulating data in molecular and cell biology and to maintain a broad experience with the social and psychological aspects of medicine.

2

The Physician in Practice

If the physician's importance to society had depended on an ability to reverse or materially alter the progress of disease, society would have dispensed with doctors centuries ago. The fact is, however, that in all societies over the range of known history the medicine man has been heavily relied upon despite the paucity of his resources with which to reverse or materially affect the progress of disease. For many centuries he had only his own "magic," his authority, dedication, and spirit. Now, with more impressive weapons with which to protect his fellow man from the ravages of disease, most physicians are "too busy" to devote time to understanding their patients as people. Perhaps our concern with the technology of medicine has made us less aware of the healing force of a genuine interest in the patient.

The Technological Imperative in Medicine

There is a wonderful story about Dr. Melvin Cassberg, one-time vice president of the University of Texas. As an avid fisherman he was trying out a river in India famous for good fishing. He hired an Indian boatman and his rowboat and into it he piled the latest and fanciest fishing gear and eagerly put it to use. After hours of casting and moving about the river without catching a fish, Cassberg was clearly discouraged. The old boatman, feeling sorry for the professor, quietly guided the boat close to a school of fish. Suddenly grabbing a net from the bottom of the boat, he threw it over the school, quickly tightened the purse, drew the net full of fish aboard and dumped them before the astounded Cassberg. "Well sir," said the boatman apologetically, "when you don't have the best equipment you have to use your head." Cassberg's failure was not due to deficiencies in the equipment but to his having overlooked an important determinant of successful fishing, proximity of the fish.

It has become fashionable to put the blame for inadequate attention to the patient's story and to the physical examination on rapid advances in the sciences basic to medicine, and especially on the growing profusion of technological tools. One adherent of this view, John Dawson, Director of the British Medical Association wrote as follows:

> Only the 'hands-on' physician might survive automation's march on medical practice by the end of this century with internists, psychiatrists, and other specialists, who rely on intellectual judgement, gradually fading. (Dawson, 1982)

A similar pessimistic view was held by Robert Moser, who, when speaking to the American Clinical and Climatological Association in 1979, suggested that the gifted bedside teacher, skilled at eliciting and evaluating evidence while communicating with and examining his patient, is rapidly becoming an anachronism (Moser, 1979). Perhaps they have read the tea leaves correctly, but I will wager that if the thinking doctor is an endangered species, neither science nor technology is responsible, but a variety of other factors including the frantic competitive arena from which medical students are selected, and the decline in the available opportunities for independent reasoning during their medical education.

Perhaps the first major technological development, now indispensable to medicine, was made by Antony van Leeuwenhoek (1633–1723) with his invention of the microscope. Interestingly, he published most of his microscopic discoveries in the *Philosophical Transactions of the Royal Society of London*. The account of his discovery of capillaries, however, was not accepted for publication (van Leeuwenhoek, 1960). Perhaps because of this, the discovery became associated with his contemporary, Marcello Malpighi (1628–1694) who was one of the first to use van Leeuwenhoek's invention (Malpighi, 1661).

Another signal contribution was diagnostic percussion discovered by Leopold von Auenbrugger (1722–1809) in 1766. He introduced it as follows:

> I here present the reader with a new sign I have discovered for detecting diseases of the chest. This consists in the percussion of the human thorax, whereby, according to the character of the particular sound thence elicited, an opinion is formed of the internal state of that cavity. In making public my discoveries respecting this matter, I have been actuated neither by an itch for writing, nor a fondness for

speculation, but by the desire of submitting to my brethren the fruits of seven years' observation and reflexion. In doing so, I have not been unconscious of the dangers I must encounter; since it has always been the fate of those who have illuminated or improved the arts and sciences by their discoveries, to be beset by envy, malice, hatred, detraction, and calumny.

As it turned out, he was not attacked or punished, but his book met a cool reception until it was translated into French by Baron Jean Nicolas Corvisart des Marets (1755–1821) (Corvisart, 1960), a prominent exponent of clinical skills.

Of comparable significance was the invention of the stethoscope by René Théophile-Hyacinthe Laënnec (1781–1826), who published his *De L'auscultation Mediate* in 1834 (Laënnec, 1834). Soon such aids, intended to strengthen the power of the human senses, were succeeded by nonsentient technological devices. In 1895 the physicist, Wilhelm Konrad Röentgen, introduced x-rays. One unfortunate consequence of this device was that a few years later some physicians, even those in major teaching centers began to abandon percussion and auscultation, relying only on x-rays until it became apparent that x-rays cannot hear. There are useful signs in the chest that percussion and auscultation can transmit but that x-ray cannot detect.

Less than half a century after Laënnec's discovery, and less than twenty years before the introduction of the electrocardiograph, the famous French physiologist, Etienne Jules Marey (1830–1904) found a way to visualize the heartbeat. He produced a device capable of recording the potentials of the heartbeat by connecting zinc sulfate electrodes on the skin of the chest to a Lippmann electrometer and measuring the potential with a mercury column. Data from this device led Marey to discover the refractory period of the heart muscle. Marey had studied with Carl Ludwig (1816–1895) in Leipzig, the inventor of the kymograph and many other important devices. Marey went on to become the leading developer of instruments for biomedical research in France.

The origin of the electrocardiograph is well told by Emmanuel Stein, in his excellent textbook (Stein, 1976). In 1903, Professor Willem Einthoven completed the first electrocardiograph. He used a string galvanometer in which a very fine quartz fiber, coated with silver to make it electrically conductive, was stretched between the piles of a powerful electromagnet. The string underwent variable displacement when the unamplified currents arising from a patient passed through it. When it was illuminated by a very bright arc lamp beam, its shadow was focused onto a moving photographic plate. A rotary-spoked wheel was used to interrupt the beam at regular intervals to provide timing markers on the plate. Einthoven communicated details of his invention to Horace Darwin (later Sir Horace Darwin, F.R.S.) of the Cambridge Scientific Instrument Company in England, and to the Messrs. Edelmann in Germany, with a suggestion that they should design and manufacture, under royalty agreement, an "Electrocardiograph" that could be marketed. A disagreement between Einthoven and the Edelmann resulted in Einthoven working exclusively with Cambridge, who manufactured their first machine in 1911. It was delivered to a budding young British cardiologist, Dr. Thomas Lewis (1881–1945) of the University College Hospital, London. He was later knighted and became one of the world's leading heart researchers. Before 1916, eighty-seven Cambridge electrocardiographs had been manufactured and shipped to fifteen countries as far distant as Japan, Australia, India, and Russia. In 1911, Dr. Horatio B. Williams of the United States visited Einthoven and, upon his return, built an instrument with Charles Hindle, his mechanic. Hindle established a manufacturing company in New York State and merged with the British firm, Cambridge Instrument Company, Ltd., in 1922, changing its name to Cambridge Instrument Company, Inc. Since then, both American and British firms have benefited from their continuing exchange of new technologies.

Marey continued his interest in visual devices. He found himself one summer morning peering at a flock of birds flying above him. He had had an interest in aerodynamics for several years and even had dreamed of building a flying machine. Suddenly, it occurred to him that the rotating chamber principle of the British Gatling gun could be applied to photographic film, and that rapidly photographing a bird as it flew could provide a rapid sequence of pictures that would then yield a "moving" picture of the flight. Apart from forwarding the science of aerodynamics, Marey's discovery led to the development of motion pictures (Marey, 1886). One of his students Joachim Carvallo, using the same gattling gun principle, developed a device comparable to the yet-to-be-invented fluoroscope by taking a series of several x-ray images of the contractions of the stomach (Carvallo, 1902).[1]

Anesthesia and bacteriology made their appearance and were followed by other technological improvements that we could not do without. The products of engineering such as needles, cannulae, and syringes were devised and perfected to the point of being indispensable. Clinical thermometry, blood counts, and chemical analyses were not far behind. Since World War II a vast array of technological developments has done much to sharpen diagnostic ability and to delay death, sometimes for many years.

As the various imaging techniques, ultrasound, radioactive tracers, immune and genetic markers, and other high-tech developments have become more and more heavily relied on, as mentioned earlier, some present-day practitioners fail to pay close attention to the medical history and physical examination. Both are indispensable sources of crucial information in the diagnosis and treatment of the patient. Neither x-rays nor imaging can speak for the patient or convey sounds from the heart or chest or give the doctor direct access to the person in the patient. It is likely, therefore, that conscientious physicians will come to realize that no technical diagnostic device, including computers, can obtain some kinds of crucially important information from a patient with nearly the power of a skillful personal dialogue.

Understanding the Patient

The need to understand the patient as a person was well stated by David P. Barr, in his presidential address to the American College of Physicians 35 years ago. He perceived that the causation of the illness is clearly non-linear and partly dependent on potentially pathogenic personal and environmental circumstances that an effective clinician needs to know about. He further warned against making diagnoses and decisions without consideration of personal problems, interpersonal family relationships, and community occupation (Barr, 1955). We might hear it better from Plato, Barr added:

> ...so neither ought you to attempt to cure the body without the soul; and this is the reason why the cure of many diseases is unknown to the physicians of Hellas, because they are ignorant of the whole which ought to be studied also; for the part can never be well unless the whole is well.... For this is the great error of our day in the treatment of the human body, that physicians separate the soul from the body.

An additional and important feature of the "whole patient" concept is the awareness that organ systems do not become disrupted in disease as separate units but as members of a widespread system of physiological inter-actions regulated by the brain and responsive to environmental forces of all sorts, including personal relationships and other life experiences. It is no accident that the earliest physicians were also priests. Whether prac-ticed in an ivory tower or at the crossroads, medicine must concern itself with the patient's adjustment to life. A physician, part philosopher and part scientist, must learn to take the artisan aspects of his practice in his stride and not hold them as his central concern.

No matter what his specialty may be, the doctor who cares for pa-tients must meet other stiff requirements, starting with certain personal qualifications that include an interest in patients and the willingness and skill to understand people and their problems. The physician needs equa-nimity to tolerate a patient's displaced hostility felt toward parents, spouse, or boss. The physician also needs equanimity to tolerate his or her own anxiety and to convey support and encouragement while the patient is slowly working through misinterpretations and poor decisions toward a better adjustment. He or she must also be prepared to worry along with little progress or settle for a limited objective, realizing that rejecting the patient or giving him up as a bad job would be destructive. Finally, the physician needs restraint. He must be particularly careful not to express contempt, ridicule, or disapproval directly or indirectly by word or ges-ture. He must avoid pressing a course of action that the patient may not be able or ready to accept, however obvious it may seem to the physi-cian. Especially, he must assiduously avoid unconsciously using his pa-tient to work out his own problems and conflicts or dominating the patient to enhance his or her own feeling of security.

The physician, therefore, needs experience in psychiatry in order prop-erly to approach and interview a patient. He or she should learn the sig-nificance of blocking, of projections, of associations, and so on. Just as a physician must know the signs of digitalis intoxication, he or she must know the signs of overexploration, evidence of impending panic, disor-ganization, or serious depression. These signs are recognizable, reason-ably clear-cut, and are just as readily learned by inquisitive medical students as are the signs of overdosage of a drug. Therefore, dealing with the person in the patient is a must for any physician or surgeon regard-less of his or her area of specialization.

It is not fashionable these days to speak of bedside manner. The fa-mous painting by Luke Fildes showing the doctor in a vigil beside the

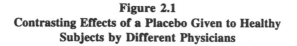

Figure 2.1
Contrasting Effects of a Placebo Given to Healthy
Subjects by Different Physicians

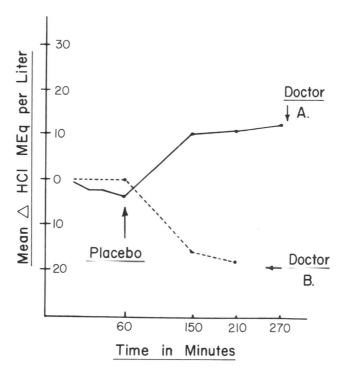

bed of a sick little girl is nowadays taken to suggest the erstwhile impotence of medicine in the face of serious infection. We seem to have made a complete substitution of miracle drugs and technology for the almost miraculous personal influence of the doctor. From the standpoint of the patient, it is a poor swap. I remember a remark by the president of the Oklahoma State Medical Society, made in the early 1950s when tranquilizers were just coming in. He said he was opposed to them because they were being used as an alternative to the doctor's dialogue with the patient, a dialogue that would enable him to know and to understand his patient. The speaker, a urologist, recognized the therapeutic quality of the person of the physician.

In treatment of any disorder, the behavior of the physician will weigh heavily in the balance. A pill, potion or even a surgical procedure administered with enthusiasm and with the promise of hope has its greatest chance of success. The physiologic consequences of human interactions are vividly illustrated by a placebo experiment we did several years ago. Opposite effects were obtained when a placebo was administered by different individuals on separate occasions to a group of medical students (figure 2.1). Such results tell us something of the dynamics of the doctor-patient relationship. Similarly bed rest, diet and others of our therapeutic rituals owe a part of their success to the quality of the communication between physician and patient.

The Dialogue

The essence of the art of medicine is expressed in the physician's dialogue with the patient. The first requirement is a genuinely earnest and sympathetic interest in the patient as a person. The patient must be encouraged to confide whatever doubts and conflicts he may care to discuss as the physician listens without implication of judgment or censure. There is much to attest that the reassurance and emotional support for the patient that stem from the physician's attitude of concerned interest and acceptance may be the most powerful psychotherapeutic tools available. Attempting by various means to uncover repressions and induce the patient to reorient his or her attitude toward people and events is an undertaking that usually requires special technical training. The physician who is not a technical specialist, however, may accomplish a great deal if he or she is dependable and engenders sufficient confidence to make it possible for the patient to express bottled-up hostilities and to deal constructively with feelings of guilt. It is equally essential to give serious and attentive consideration to all bodily symptoms, even though no explanation may be offered and no medication given for them. Much damage can be done by "brushing off" or being impatient with a person's complaints. An explanation of the psychological and bodily mechanisms that underlie symptoms may be helpful but should not be "pushed" if the patient does not readily accept it. It is especially unwise to force the patient to "insight" to induce him to acknowledge a connection between his personal conflicts and his symptoms. Very often a patient will deny such a relationship, and yet, paradoxically, will talk freely as if he were aware of the connection. This "face saving" screen is frequently very important to the patient. There is often little to be gained and much to be

lost by breaking it down. The physician can sometimes help in the resolution of dilemmas and to mitigate the doubts and conflicts of indecision
by helping the patient learn that the solution of serious problems is
achieved neither by side-stepping nor blind confrontation, but rather by
a carefully thought out strategy for dealing with them constructively.
Thus, the physician often functions as a teacher. "Teacher" is the literal
meaning of doctor. Effective teaching demands a sensitive awareness of
clues and alertness to opportunities as they emerge from time to time in a
discussion. Illuminating his observed concerns may enable the patient to
arrive at a satisfactory resolution of his dilemma or to reach a decision
with which he can live.

"Subtractive" Surgery

Several years ago Dr. Arthur Sutherland showed that deprivation by
surgery of bodily members or organs commonly resulted in serious
psychologic difficulties that often went unrecognized by the patients'
physicians and surgeons. He found that the loss of an organ, as from
amputations, plastic procedures, and, most important of all, colostomy,
often impair a patient's self-esteem or his or her feeling of acceptability
by family or friends. Sutherland pointed out that, because many intelli-
gent patients have such a poor knowledge of anatomy, they are likely to
conjure up weird and fanciful impressions of the results of surgery. After
surgery many of his colostomy patients became so compulsive as to be
incapacitated by the ritual of cleaning and caring for the bowel. Some
spent as much as eight hours a day in the bathroom carrying out irriga-
tions and other procedures with the colostomy.

Sutherland showed that many of the problems of postoperative reha-
bilitation could be avoided by simply discussing with the patient, prior to
operation, the nature of the postoperative handicap and the possibilities
for adjustment. In fact, he found strikingly close correlation of smooth
postoperative recovery with who said what to the patient on the evening
before the surgery (Sutherland, 1952). The least favorable recoveries
were in those patients who had not been visited by any of the staff on the
evening prior to operation. The best results were observed when the surgeon who was to operate, had visited and brought his reassurance. Then,
in decreasing degree favorable results related to a preliminary visit from
the referring physician, the anesthesiologist, the head nurse, or another

nurse. Even a cheerful visit from one of the housekeepers was apparently of some help toward a reasonably comfortable recovery.

It is especially helpful if the surgeon is aware of the role the body part about to be removed plays in the general life adjustment of this patient— what its meaning and importance are to the individual. If the patient is allowed to develop a firm, sympathetic, and trusting relationship with his surgeon, he can tolerate subtractive surgery better than he can if he is merely given explanations. When the surgeon is "too busy" to allow a suitable relationship to develop with his patient, the physician must assume the task of educating the patient and preparing him emotionally for operation. Thus, beyond the great benefits realized from technical progress, there is much that close attention to the person in the patient can tell us that we may ignore to our jeopardy and to that of the patient. Sutherland's work probably had a good deal to do with the organization of mutual patient support groups such as ostomy clubs.

The Dying Patient

As advances in medicine have disposed of some old problems, they have created new ones for the practitioner. Antibiotics, antimetabolites and numerous mechanical devices have not only prolonged life but have prolonged dying as well. Lobar pneumonia, Osler's "friend of the old people," which once mercifully carried off the hopelessly ill, has been all but eliminated. Thus, today more than ever, a major responsibility of the physician is caring for the hopeless, the dying, a responsibility that calls for a special knowledge of the ways of the world and a sensitivity to, and understanding of, suffering people.

The physician needs to know each of his patients as a person so that at the bedside of the dying he may make the proper individualized judgments. Some patients prefer to die alone, others with their families about them. Some would prefer to be so narcotized as to be unaware of their fading life, while others prefer the awareness of life as long as it lasts. The decision as to how to handle the situation is therefore made on the basis of the physician's knowledge of his patient's personality. He must enlist the cooperation of family, the nurses, and other ward personnel to follow a consistent plan that will provide the greatest comfort for the patient. The comfort of the dying is rarely contributed to by an atmosphere of hectic application of heroic last-minute, would-be life-saving measures such as transfusions and infusions and other needle therapy, oxygen tents, and pulmotors. On the other hand, it may be discouraging to a patient for the physician suddenly to clear the room of such devices in anticipation of death. The most important thing is for the physician to communicate with his patient so that he can help him with what he wants and needs most during his last hours. It is rarely necessary to talk much, but it is extremely important to listen and to be aware of communications other than verbal ones. The strength and ability of the patient to meet the terminal phase of life depend on those circumstances that strengthen his courage and faith, including a trusting and supportive relationship with his doctor. Therefore, rather than keeping the patient at arm's length, rather than making light of the situation, rather than fooling himself that the patient is extraordinarily stoical, the physician should attempt to share the patient's experience in a dignified and steadfast way.

A human being's ability to tolerate tragedy and disaster can be greatly enhanced by the presence of a strong, understanding, and sympathetic person. Part of the job of the doctor is to share the burden. There is no place in modern medicine for the attitude of hurried austerity so popular among surgeons of a generation or two ago. At the time, while making great strides in assuaging or preventing the pain of their knives, they were causing other pains often less bearable and longer lasting.

There is always the urge to "do something," and frequently this inward urge of the physician is strongly reinforced by demands of the patient's family. The one important thing to do is to see the patient frequently, to provide him often with the reassuring presence of doctors and nurses and other members of the staff. It is also important for the doctor to speak frequently with the family, if only to tell them that there is no change, and to be available to answer their anxious questions. The key to equanimity of the dying patient and of his family is the early establishment of an interested, sympathetic relationship, giving the patient the assurance that the physician is doing his utmost and will support the patient and his family to the last.

There is abundant evidence that the nature of interpersonal communication, the influence of one person on another, the atmosphere created by an individual's personality or behavior has measurable and often powerful effects on body physiology and even pathogenic processes. While quite distinct from the currently popular high technology of medicine, the person of the doctor is a therapeutic resource of great potential value to the patient.

Nourishing the Spirit

We have finally learned that effective social adjustment that yields personal satisfaction and fulfillment is conducive to health; and that social failure, frustration, dissatisfaction, deprivation, and disapproval increase vulnerability to disease. These data are not new, but neither are they widely accepted. To achieve personal fulfillment one must approve of one's self, must find others in harmony with one's system of values. In continually electing, consciously or unconsciously, among various alternatives a certain course to pursue, we may satisfy the needs of the spirit quite apart from those for personal survival, food, and sexual gratification.

When altruism has been recognized in animal forms, including man, many psychologists and anthropologists have passed off altruistic behavior, somewhat lamely, as sick exaggerations of restraint or vicarious gratification of a basic instinct for praise. The facts of history do not really bear out such a selfish interpretation. As C.P. Snow said in *The Two Cultures and the Scientific Revolution*: "It is a mistake which anyone who is called realistic is especially liable to fall into, to think that when we have said something about the egotism, the weaknesses, the vanities, and the power-seekings of men, we have said everything, but they are sometimes capable of more. And any realism which doesn't admit of that isn't serious" (Snow, 1961).

It may be that the positive nourishment of the spirit of man contains an important key to his health and growth. It may be, indeed, that we will find that altruism is a hard, practical asset, just as cooperation turned out to be.[2] Altruism may provide a third dimension to evolution and accelerate even further man's quest for his goals. It was certainly a great discovery when animals first learned that they could protect themselves by exterminating one another. When it was learned that cooperation had more survival value than competition, a startling contribution to progress had been made. Perhaps we will learn that generosity of spirit has even more power. There is certainly widespread evidence that a person with a primary concern for the welfare of others reaps greater comfort and satisfaction than he or she would from seeking only selfish interests. Isn't this what happens when an organization has superb morale, or in the many human situations where superior teamwork wins? The ability to hope, to trust in others, the ability to have faith in one's destiny and to realize one's personal identity are the elements of emotional security that can sustain an individual through all manner of hazards and hardships. The expectations of those about us, the standards of our culture and the demands of one's particular social milieu are powerful forces, now driving, now restraining, that may either threaten or sustain a person.

As social demands and preferences vary from nation to nation, or from one enclave to another in a large American city, the forces that shape character, behavior, and sensitivities of the inhabitants may differ widely. For example, from my experience in New York City I learned that children from Italian families were often characteristically faced with a severe emotional challenge at around eighteen years of age. Up to then the girls had been sheltered by their parents against any lengthy association with boys. In fact, a father would often keep track of the time his daughter took to return home from school. Then, when she reached eighteen, he would express surprise that she was not yet engaged to be married. At eighteen, the boys with Italian parents were encouraged to "get a good job." Their parents tended to downplay aspirations for higher education, or even advanced technical training.

One of my patients, an Italian-American, had hoped to become an engineer. His best friend and neighbor, a Jewish boy, had been urged by his mother to work hard to become a doctor, lawyer, or engineer, and she was willing to assume the necessary financial sacrifices to make it possible for him. The boy, however, did not share her aspirations and simply wanted to "get a good job." Both boys eventually developed chronic peptic ulcer. These and other familiar experiences, suggest that physicians should be aware of the social forces that impinge on individual patients in their care. Had the physicians in these cases taken into account the powerful significance of social and family traditions and parental pressures, they would have realized that effectively treating a patient with peptic ulcer requires far more than a parietal cell blocker and an antibiotic.

Social customs and family traditions are not necessarily stress producing. They may, on the other hand, be strongly supportive of the aspirations of the youth, especially regarding education. This was true of the inhabitants of a closely knit Italian American community, Roseto, Pennsylvania, established more than 100 years ago and discussed below.

The Power of Social Support

The town of Roseto in eastern Pennsylvania was found to be remarkably healthy and comparatively free of the major scourges in America such as cardiovascular and mental illness. The death rate from myocardial infarction in this almost exclusively Italian town of 1,700 inhabitants, was less than half that of surrounding towns (Bruhn & Wolf, 1979). Roseto was originally settled in 1882 by immigrants from Roseto Val Fortore in the province of Foggia in Italy. The town became the subject of careful study for thirty years beginning in 1962. The conventional risk factors for myocardial infarction were by no means absent among Rosetans. We found that a diet high in animal fat, cigarette smoking, relatively sedentary occupation, and obesity, are at least as prevalent in Roseto as elsewhere in the northeastern part of the United States. Neither could the comparatively salubrious state of Rosetans be attributed to genetic or ethnic factors. A study of their relatives, many born in Roseto, who now live in towns and cities in New York, New Jersey, and Pennsylvania areas, revealed stigmata of coronary artery disease by history and electrocardiogram comparable to other Americans. Moreover, their families had suffered the usual number of deaths from myocardial infarction among men in the fourth and fifth decades. In Roseto, on the other hand, only one individual had died of myocardial infarction under the age of fifty-five. The striking feature of Roseto was its social structure. Because the Italians had been shunned by the mainly Anglo-Saxon inhabitants of the region, their natural cohesiveness was actually accentuated. Not only were the family units extremely close and mutually supportive, but so was the community as a whole, so that there was essentially no poverty and virtually no crime. The male-female relationships in Roseto were those of the "old country" with the man the undisputed head of the household. The aged in Roseto retained their position of influence in the family and in the community. They were kept in the home, cherished, respected, and were turned to, like a supreme court, for the solution of family problems.

In contrast to the social mores in Roseto were those of Nazareth, Pennsylvania just twelve miles away. Nazareth, one of the communities in the vicinity that was studied as a control, was settled in 1740 by the Moravians, a strict religious group from southern Germany.[3] There, senior citizens were expected to pass on the torch of leadership to their young middle-aged sons. In fact, the first "old folks" home in the United States was established in Nazareth. It is a prosperous and conservative community inhabited mainly by people of German descent. The prevalence of coronary disease and the death rate from myocardial infarction in Nazareth was closely similar to that in the U.S. at large.

In addition to their relative immunity from death due to myocardial infarction, we found, among the people of Roseto a remarkably low incidence of mental illness, especially senile dementia (Bruhn & Wolf, 1970). Roseto has taught us that social stability and mobility are not necessarily antithetical. Like a ship underway, the community was stable with respect to certain buffetings and yet moved forward. Thus, Roseto was economically prosperous in comparison to its neighbors and innovative with respect to community projects. Thanks to the leadership of Father Denisco a highly educated and determined priest, who played the role of community leader during the town's early days, education had a high priority among the Italians of Roseto. By the time we studied the community in 1962, most of Roseto's high school entrants went on to graduation and an unusually high percentage of them completed a four-year college course.

We were eventually able to test our hypothesis that the relative immunity to coronary deaths among Rosetans was related to their culture. From interviews with Rosetans under thirty years of age in 1962, we predicted that, with a loosening of family solidarity and failure to adhere to the old world values that had served them well since their immigration in 1882, they would lose their relative immunity to fatal heart attack. After a few years we noted that the pattern of "old country" cohesiveness had begun to weaken. The younger people were not identifying themselves with the community activities to the extent they formerly did. They were even joining country clubs and attending church outside of Roseto. Their attitudes were becoming more typical of the prevailing culture in the communities around them.

In a reexamination and reevaluation of the population twenty-three years later, we learned not only that rapid and dramatic social changes had taken place, but that, as predicted, the death rate from myocardial infarction had increased progressively and had matched that of the neighboring towns that we had been studying as controls (Wolf & Bruhn, 1993).

Dr. Sula Benet, a professor of anthropology at Hunter College, New York, reported among the Abkhasians of Georgia in the USSR a salubrious social pattern comparable to the earlier pattern we observed in Roseto. She wrote of their remarkable health and longevity, emphasizing "the high degree of integration in their lives, the sense of group identity that gives each individual an unshaken feeling of personal security and continuity and permits the Abkhasians as a people to adapt themselves—yet preserve themselves—to the changing conditions imposed by the larger society in which they live." Also in common with Roseto, and in contrast to most American communities, the place of the elderly in the community of Abkhasians was very special. Dr. Benet wrote that as "a life-loving, optimistic people, [they are] unlike so many old 'dependent' people in the United States who feel they are burdens to themselves and their families...they enjoy the prospect of continued life.... In a culture that so highly values continuity in its traditions, the old are indispensable in their transmission. The elders preside at important ceremonial occasions, they mediate disputes and their knowledge of farming is sought. They feel needed because...they are" (Benet, 1965).

The challenge for modern society is to preserve, insofar as possible, the salubrious influence of established patterns in the face of inevitable and increasingly rapid change. Another important requirement of individuals in a healthy society is their constructive interdependence, a fundamental principle governing the health and welfare of living creatures. The realization of this truth may have been somewhat obscured by Darwin's emphasis on competition, the survival of the fit. It is true, nevertheless, that interdependence is demonstrable in the simplest of unicellular organisms. The top millimeter of the sea, for example, is occupied by a variety of microscopic forms, each separate and freely moving, but the product of one is essential to the life of another so that these unconnected cells are nevertheless very closely interrelated. Such interdependent aggregations must be the forerunners of tissues. It appears, therefore, that the process of nature has been differentiation, specialization, combination, and then differentiation again. There may be a great lesson for us in the story of interdependence. Perhaps cities are the tissue of human society. The mass of humanity on the face of the earth may be comparable to the organisms in the top millimeter of the sea. The interrelatedness of all life, and hence the identity of life above and apart from individual identity, is expressed by Teilhard de Chardin in this concept of the biosphere, which is ever changing and evolving (Teilhard de Chardin, 1955).

The ability of individuals to achieve healthy relationships and to ac-
commodate to change depends on the plasticity of the nervous system—
that is, on the ability to alter functional connections between association
neurons and to make selections among pathways of behavior. It is tempt-
ing, therefore, to speculate that the often proposed relationship of self-
esteem, self-confidence, and optimism to health has a sound scientific
basis.

There is ample evidence that the nourishment of the spirit is relevant
to bodily health and performance. At Western Electric, when the company officials wanted to find out whether fluorescent lighting would increase the efficiency of working women, they installed it in one of the
workrooms. The productivity of the group working in that room soon
exceeded the productivity of all other groups. Then it was suggested that
the women might do even better if the walls were painted a pastel shade.
That worked, too. Really interested by now, the management decided to
test the effect of increasing the height of the workbenches by six inches.
Again productivity increased, but then it was discovered that lowering
the workbenches six inches had the same effect. Ultimately, it became
clear to the officials that what was helping these workers toward better
achievement was the recognition that someone was interested in their
welfare and comfort.

Another famous experiment was carried out by Frederick the Great in
a foundling hospital in Germany (Gooch, 1990). To cut down the mortality rate by eliminating germs, insofar as possible, he ordered the hospital attendants to change the babies' linen frequently, to keep things
scrupulously clean, and to feed the children promptly but without holding or cuddling them in any way. Thus he hoped to avoid communicable
diseases. Surprisingly, however, the lack of human warmth and loving
resulted in the death of most of the babies, although at autopsy there
were no specific lesions discernible.

How often have we seen the broken spirit of an aged person lead to his
deterioration and death when he no longer felt wanted or useful. Dr.
Calvin Plimpton, the president of Amherst College, tells the story of a
man who died and shortly thereafter found himself transported to a de-
lightfully cool and comfortable spot where his every want was supplied
as soon as he mentioned it. In fact, one of the angels, who appeared to be
assigned to him, continually asked him what he would like to have in
order to raise his level of enjoyment. He asked for, and received, a fine

house with a kidney-shaped swimming pool, a fine car, and a few fine young ladies, as well as a few rather prosaic luxuries. He was having difficulty in deciding just what else he desired, when one day he asked, "Isn't there some work I could do around here?" The angel replied, "Oh, gracious, no! There's no work." "Well, couldn't I be useful in some way? Isn't there something I could help out with?" There seemed to be no opportunities along this line at all. Becoming more and more restless, the man kept imploring the angel for some little thing he might undertake in the way of work, but always with the same reply. Finally, in exasperation he said, "Well, if it's going to go on like this indefinitely, I would have preferred to go to Hell." "And just where," said the angel, "do you think you are?" (Plimpton, 1960).

The study of the lofty aspects of man's spirit ought to prove as interesting and as fruitful as the study of his more earthy qualities. In fact, this might be the new frontier for psychiatry.

Notes

1. The Gatling gun, consisting of a revolving cluster of loaded barrels around a central core, was actually invented by an American, R.J. Gathney, (1818–1903). Carvallo's invention was made in 1903, seven years after W.C. Roentgen's discovery of the x-ray.
2. Wise men over the ages have extolled the importance of altruism to civilization. An early philosopher, Mencius (372–289 B.C.) wrote: "Benevolence is the tranquil habitation of man, and righteousness is his straight path." (Works, bk. 2, 1:10.2 from *The Chinese Classics, 1861–1886*, vol. II, The works of Mencius, translated by James Legge).
3. The Protestant religion of the Moravians was founded by Jan Hus from a small group known as Unitas Fratrem Fratres Bohemiae. Count Nicholas, Ludwig von Zinzendorf in 1740–41, established a Moravian community in Nazareth and Bethlehem, Pennsylvania. Bethlehem became the center of trade and industry, while Nazareth remained an agricultural community. No one was paid wages. Instead, everyone became one household and worked for the good of the whole. The church owned all the land, buildings, and tools. Bishop Spangenburg and his wife headed what was known as the General Economy. They presided over the committees that managed the details of government.

3

Medicine in Relation to Society

The Expectations of Society

For centuries, in order to maintain their military, political, and economic strength, nations have concerned themselves with the health of their people. Such justifications are still cogent today, but modern philosophy places an equal emphasis on individual fulfillment and well-being, an emphasis that is likely to become stronger over the next few decades.

The course of history has changed as man, always striving to satisfy his needs, has perceived them differently from time to time. There has also been a cumulative effect over the years so that he has progressively demanded more and more of his environment. This development, and the fact that man himself has contributed mightily to changes in his environment, has helped to bring about increasing interdependence among people, an interdependence that stretches across greater and greater distances. Thus a concern for the welfare of other individuals and groups, and even more or less remote nations, is no longer purely a matter of altruism. As recognized by the learned presidential advisor Adolph Berle, this concern contributes quite directly to one's own safety and welfare (Berle, 1963). Perhaps increasing interdependence, as an aspect of the evolution of man, might be called a natural law of society.

The evolution of society has owed much to man's continual curiosity, his relentless inquiry into the laws of nature, and particularly into the laws that govern man himself. Increasing knowledge of these has enabled him to define more clearly his basic needs. Where he used to see food and shelter as essential elements, he now expects comfort and security, health and medical care. It is pertinent to ask what may reasonably be required of the health professions over the coming years. The naive and thoughtless may ask for freedom from illness and indefinitely postponed death, conditions we can confidently omit from any realistic anticipation. Death, after all, is a part of life, a necessary condition to biological or even social evolution. A greater number of people may live longer as the scourges of youth and middle age are mitigated, but there is little likelihood that more than the occasional hearty human will come near to spanning a century. Individual illnesses may be conquered but, as René Dubos showed so beautifully in his *Mirage of Health*, as we tamper with the environment new patterns of disease appear to challenge the ingenuity of medical science (Dubos, 1959).

The American public has been bombarded with spectacular stories of scientific advances and with propaganda of all sorts concerning medical and health care, but nevertheless much of the public remains naive concerning their fundamental needs and the real potential of the medical establishment. Today the primary concern of most laymen with respect to their health needs is availability of physicians. Their second concern is a method of payment. Most Americans, especially in rural and semirural areas, want reasonable access to a physician, and preferably a choice of physicians. The standard usually quoted for the proper distribution of physicians per population density, one physician for every 1,000 patients, is based on the transportation and communication systems that prevailed at the turn of the century.

Despite problems of geography, health needs are certainly being provided for more effectively now than in the past. Interest in preventive medicine has followed the elimination or neutralization of microbes and other noxious agents, the focus has shifted to the host, his innate adaptive capacities, and his individual proclivities. Developmental studies are also proceeding on a broad front. Pediatricians and psychiatrists have been studying the formative years from birth through adolescence for clues to the possibility of shaping the individual into a more adaptable, healthier adult.

As physicians become increasingly effective in dealing with the broad spectrum of disorders and diseases, the public will grow increasingly aware of its needs and its due. Since man is continually creating new hazards to health, the medical establishment will be expected to provide for the health needs of everyone at a price everyone can afford. It follows that new measures must be devised to bring the best of medical and health care within reach. In a search for solutions, businessmen, insurance agents, and legislators have been busily developing health care plans.

No plan, of course, and no organization for distribution of services will of itself insure proper quality. Much more is involved than managerial efficiency and financial feasibility. Quality of medical care ultimately depends on the personal characteristics and education of physicians and other health personnel.

The Challenge

Although the epidemics that once decimated whole communities have largely been conquered and while in our part of the world, at least, we have been made relatively secure from hunger and homelessness, man is not happy, not fulfilled. Neither is he particularly healthy. Repeatedly, over the course of recorded history, his preoccupation with material comforts and conveniences has, like an unbalanced diet, somehow sickened him. His education and experiences, have not yet taught him that his health and well-being depend, not only on his capacity to adapt to the tangible environment, but also to prevailing attitudes and values in his society and to his own goals and aspirations.

There are now at least some indications that the man of Western civilization is becoming aware of his state of spiritual and emotional starvation.[1] As he does, more and more will be required of the physician. Not only will he need to be a capable diagnostician who knows his limitations and operates within them, but a counselor of some intellectual quality, wisdom, and experience as well. He will have to supplement a broad knowledge, analytical judgment, and experience with disease with an understanding of people and of the forces, tangible and symbolic, with which they must deal. He will apply his knowledge that the bodily organs and tissues are subject to a complex system of controls, a hierarchy in which precedence is taken by impulses from the highest integrative levels of the brain, those areas concerned with the interpretation of experience. He will possess an interest in people as individuals and a respect for their individuality. In short, the modern physician will effectively serve the people by offering them informed, comprehensive, and continuing care.

Medical educators and their parent universities share with the practicing profession the responsibility for the future of American medicine, responsibility for guiding their students and institutions toward meeting the health needs of tomorrow. This means bringing the best of medical and health care ever closer to the people in a changing society. If the desired state is to be reached, both town and gown must be sensitive to the currents of history and the changing needs of the people, as river pilots are to the special characteristics of the channel. Individually and collectively, practitioners and academicians must examine their values and objectives, assessing the significance of and justification for conflicts where they exist among them because ultimately the goal of the whole medical establishment, to care for people, is a common one.

The Social Sciences and Medicine

The social sciences might be thought of as those disciplines that concern themselves with man's relationship to man. Inevitably then, they deal with human values—aims, goals, and attitudes, conscious and unconscious. Thus the social sciences deal with the highest integrative functions of the human nervous system. Presumably, the high development of the mammalian nervous system has been responsible for our continued presence in the world. The dinosaurs had far more formidable weapons of attack and defense than did the mammals, and yet they became extinct about the time the mammalian design was developed in the course of evolution.

Although mammals were generally more vulnerable than reptiles, they were also more adaptable. The integrative activity of their brains provided for maintaining the temperature of their blood more or less constant in the face of variations of 100 degrees or more in the surrounding atmosphere. Mammals also were able to adapt to wetness and dryness, to altitudes, and to the wily predatory maneuvers of their enemies. It would appear, therefore, that the purpose of the brain may be stated not so much in terms of maintaining constancy of the internal environment but rather of providing effective adaptations to change in both the internal and external environments, including changes in social pressures, hazards, and challenges (Wolf, 1961).

Important adjustments to cultural and social pressures and to interpersonal stresses are made through the interpretive areas of the brain. The social scientist has a good deal to contribute to education in clinical medicine and neuroscience.

It might be fair to say that until recently the social sciences stood in relation to medicine where chemistry did 150 years ago. In 1847 Rudolf Virchow observed: "Chemistry has already accomplished a great deal for us, although thus far very little is useful for practical purposes. We expect a great deal more from it" (Virchow, 1958). At that early time Virchow recognized not only the importance of chemistry, but the importance of social science to medicine. In his own words: "Medicine is a social science in its very bone and marrow" (Virchow, 1958). He was proposing that the problems of the state be placed in the hands of medical scientists whom he considered to be most familiar with the social, as well as biological nature of man and his needs. We have been slow to act on Virchow's broad insight.[2]

Parkinson, referring to the continued failure of educators to recognize the significance of technological developments in social terms offered the following:

> When the moment comes to launch the space ship the equipment used will represent the latest thing in technical and scientific progress. The scientists in charge of the operation will be the leaders (we hope) in their respective fields of knowledge. All that is obsolete by contrast will be represented on the platform. There under the awning and between the potted plants will be grouped the politicians, the party chiefs, the religious spokesmen, the venerated community leaders and the accepted prophets of the age and they will all be completely and utterly out of touch with the matter in hand. They will typify the government, the directing body and all that is most respected in our social system, the one part of our organization which we have completely forgotten to modernize. (Parkinson, 1960)

Virchow's idea was perhaps much like Parkinson's. In 1849 Virchow wrote:

> If medicine is the science of the healthy as well as the ill human being, what other science is better suited to propose laws as the basis of the social structure in order to make effective those which are inherent in man himself? Once medicine is established as anthropology and once the interests of the privileged no longer determine the course of public events, the physiologist and the practitioner will be counted among the elder statesmen who support the social structure. (Virchow, 1958)

It was as if Virchow, 150 years ago, had recognized the need to head off the circumstances described by Parkinson. Unfortunately the fulfillment of Virchow's dream has been long in coming. The pertinence of the social sciences to medicine was clearly stated in the 1930s with the publication of the book, *Civilization and Disease* by C.P. Donnison who related the prevalence of social pressures to disease (Donnison, 1938).

Donnison's book develops the idea that as man has lived in groups of increasing size, social patterns have evolved to deal with prevailing circumstances, and, over the course of history and in various parts of the world, social structures have been altered and remodeled to meet changing circumstances. When the speed of change has outrun the pace of adaptation, Donnison holds that man's internal mechanisms, mental and physical, react inappropriately and provide what he calls the basis of the diseases of civilization.

Donnison's essentially speculative conclusions have received support from evidence gathered in the last forty years indicating that the neural and hormonal mechanisms that characterize essential hypertension, the metabolic manifestations of diabetes and Graves' disease, and the gastric acid secretion of peptic ulcer may be elicited as part of a person's reaction to psychologically threatening events (Hinkle et al., 1950; Hetzel, 1964; Wolf, 1949). Such evidence, emerging from the studies of Claude Bernard, I. Pavlov, and W.B. Cannon, was extended in clinical experimental studies on human beings by Harold Wolff and a long list of his followers. The findings are summarized in his book *Stress and Disease* (1953).

Ten years after Donnison's book appeared, J.L. Halliday in England picked up the idea of the potential pathogenicity of social forces and wrote a book called *Psychosocial Medicine* (1948). Halliday argued that although it was obvious to everyone that attention to the physical environment had made possible some of the most effective public health measures—the control of typhoid fever, cholera, plague, typhus, and other infectious diseases, and more recently the control of radiation and of pathogenic chemicals in the environment—similar concern with the psychological and social environment, however appropriate, had lagged behind.

Both Donnison and Halliday saw morale, or common purpose, as the healthy integrating force in society. They both considered disease the consequence of demoralization related to social change, change too swift or too disruptive for the adaptive capacity of the social group.

L.W. Simmons and Harold Wolff, dealing with this issue in their book *Social Science in Medicine* (1954), observed that in decaying cultures anxiety-producing factors tend to outlast those that protect against or relieve anxiety.[3] Similarly René Dubos showed that vulnerability to infectious diseases may be enhanced in a setting of rapid social change (Dubos, 1951). After a lifetime of study of tuberculosis, he concluded that unsanitary conditions, crowding, poverty, and so forth were less significant in outbreaks of the disease throughout the world than what he referred to as "social disruption," rapid social change. Many other scientists have added confirmation to the concept that the quality of social adaptation is pertinent to health. Indeed, this basic proposition has cropped up repeatedly since antiquity. Nevertheless, it is still not wholly acceptable to the biomedical community, and is as yet to be incorporated into currently prevailing thought about medicine and public health.

The increasing emphasis on the significance of homeostatic mechanisms of all sorts has made it easier to accept the proposition that perturbation of an established system may set in motion a destructive chain of events. Thus, an organism adapted to past circumstances is always to some extent maladapted to new circumstances. Daniel Brunner studied oriental Jews who were immigrating to Israel and found that shortly after arrival they had practically no heart attacks. Moreover, those who died in the early years following immigration showed at autopsy practically no arteriosclerosis in their coronary vessels. Later, however, Brunner observed that the oriental Jews had begun to have coronary artery disease, myocardial infarction (heart attack), and sudden death in rapidly increasing numbers. He pointed to the extraordinarily rapid social change that had occurred among them (Brunner, 1968).

The oriental Jew, living in a tent in the desert in Africa with his wife and children, was an absolute czar of the family. Suddenly in Israel his children were thrown into school where they associated with peer groups that emphasized, as they do in this country, "doing your own thing" and freedom. Therefore, at home, instead of showing their former automatic deference and respect to their fathers, they behaved the way your children and mine do. Moreover, the wife, who in the desert had been covered up literally and figuratively, could now exploit her skills at sewing and cooking to land a job. On the job, surrounded by the ambience of women's "lib," she might also defy her husband. One does not have to be a psychiatrist to visualize the intensity of emotional stress experienced by these oriental Jewish families.

The Social Structure and Disease

Henry Sigerist has called attention to the fact that each era in the development of Western culture has been characterized by the prevalence of certain diseases (Sigerist, 1932):

It seems as though the powers that ordain the style for and stamp their impress upon a certain epoch affect even disease. The Middle Ages, for instance, were dominated by diseases of the common people—such as the plague, leprosy, and the epidemic neuroses—which appeared in the sixth to fourteenth centuries, thus outlining that period in history. In the Renaissance it was syphilis, a distinctly individualistic disease, to which no one is subject but which is acquired through a volitional act. In the discordant Baroque era the foreground is occupied by disorders that might be called deficiency diseases like camp fever, scurvy and ergotism on the one hand and on the other by those that might be called luxury diseases, gout, dropsy and hypochondriasis. During the Romantic Era, tuberculosis and chlorosis were the diseases of the productive years of life and the leading social malaise was unrequited love.

The behavior of the romantic was characterized by expressiveness and spending. In contrast, the characteristic attitude of America's earlier Calvinistic culture was dominated by the work ethic which today has given way to a desire for accumulation and self-indulgence. Our social emphasis is on the individual rather than on family and group relationships. People have always created their social climate and, in turn, have been greatly affected by it. Behavior becomes organized and systematized into social patterns, ground rules that evolve into traditions and taboos as they weave the fabric of a culture. Much as we hate to admit it, cultures are built on conformity. What we call progress comes chiefly from the breaking of traditions, from new ideas that generate new ground rules. There is something in each of us that leans in both directions— toward change, exploration, and the testing of new ideas on the one hand, and on the other, toward conformity with tradition and the stability that comes from approval of one's peers.

The current scourge in most industrialized nations is arterial disease, especially coronary artery disease and hypertension with the all too frequent consequences of stroke, myocardial infarction and sudden death. Social patterns appear to be highly relevant to all three. For example, in a thirty-year prospective study of coronary heart disease in the Italian American community of Roseto, Pennsylvania, we saw the doubling of an initially low rate of mortality from myocardial infarction during a period of rapid change in social values and behavior characterized by rising materialism and the weakening of family ties (Wolf & Bruhn, 1993).

It is fascinating that, as mentioned, Donnison found that the diseases of Western civilization—myocardial infarction, hypertension, arthritis, and so forth—were uncommon in strongly traditional societies in Africa whose stability contrasted sharply with our highly mobile Western culture.

The Challenge of Change

Hippocrates, nearly twenty-five centuries ago, reminded his contemporaries of the risk of change when he wrote "those things which one has been accustomed to for a long time, although worse than things to which one is not accustomed, usually give less disturbance" (Hippocrates, 1938). There is much evidence to suggest that social stability is conducive to health, while social change, especially rapid change, may predispose to illness. As already mentioned, René Dubos has provided vivid examples of the relevance of environment, especially social environment, to the pathogenicity of microorganisms. He called particular attention to the importance of the rate of change. Cultures differ from one another in the extent to which they limit the choices of their members and hence yield to pressures for change. Some societies, and not necessarily primitive ones, share in common the feature of extreme stability where mores are rigidly fixed and behavioral alternatives few. Thus, in parts of India, for example, during a scarcity of grain, diet may be limited to the point of starvation despite an abundance of available fish, fowl, or meat which their religion requires them to avoid.

While malnutrition, exposure, and parasitism may shorten the lives of those who live in relatively stereotyped social settings, these people appear to suffer less from the cardiovascular and digestive disorders that are so prevalent in less strictly patterned Western societies where individual choices are wider.

We are gradually learning that, in biology, the only permanent thing is change—change requiring new adaptive responses on the part of organisms, races, and species to serve their need to survive. Man's thinking brain has both aided him in his adaptations and created new challenges for him. His science and technology have provided protection from the elements and from other destructive forces in the environment. At the same time they have endowed him with power beyond the wildest dreams of the potentates of the past, they have also confronted him with new hazards of injury, accidental death, and subtler changes in the form of radiations and noxious chemicals in the air that he breathes and in the food that he eats. Man's reckless and apparently insatiable desire to explore and experiment has led him to establish a kind of mastery over the world despite his diminutive stature, the delicacy of his offspring, and his lack of natural weapons such as sharp teeth or claws. At each point along the way, the quality of his performance has reflected the validity of his values. In terms of social as well as bodily health, though, he has often been more unadapted than adapted, more sick than well. Without having to comply with the animal's rule by instinct, the human develops attitudes and values and makes choices about his behavior that deeply affect his health and longevity.

Disability and death resulting from exposure to the elements were mitigated when man sought shelter and clothing, the wild predators were fended off with arms and the microbes with public hygiene and antibiotics. Now, the illnesses related to man's own predilections and his relations with his fellow man are gaining prominence. The creation of societies required that males learn to live together without destroying each other. Now, the survival of society requires that we learn to tolerate differences in people and their points of view. The stress-fraught adaptations concerned with this step in development provide much of what is noxious in the environment of modern man. These forces combine with others with which we must concern ourselves in examining disease mechanisms. Taking due cognizance of genetic proclivities, learned patterns of response, and pressures of all sorts—tangible and otherwise—we must look for the forces that arouse and the mechanisms that modulate adaptive efforts in the body.

Thomas Holmes, a professor on the faculty of the University of Washington, made a landmark contribution to the understanding of the pathogenic effects of change. With his student and collaborator, Richard Rahe, he perfected a quantitative scale whereby one can relate emotionally significant social changes to the statistical risk of developing disease (Holmes & Rahe, 1967). Holmes and Rahe found that those whose lives had been disrupted to some extent by major events such as the death of a spouse or the loss of a job, and even by less dramatic changes such as assuming a financial debt or taking a vacation, were at increased risk of illness of all sorts. The various "life changes," as they were called, were rated as to their potential significance. The Holmes and Rahe scale has been applied to several different cultures and nationalities around the globe, and has been found generally reliable as a predictor of susceptibility to illness.

Despite the potential health hazards of change it may, nevertheless, be as essential to growth for individuals as it is for social systems. The challenge, then is to learn to adapt to inevitable change.

Medical Implications of Social Change in Brunei, Borneo

A few years ago I had an opportunity to observe adaptation in a community undergoing rapid change. I joined the cruise of the Scripps research vessel, *Alpha Helix*, to Brunei, in north Borneo, where my son, Tom, and I studied the effects of rapid social change in rural tribes dwelling in jungle communities (Wolf & Wolf, 1978). For about 10,000 years and until oil was discovered on the shore of Brunei, very little change in social patterns seems to have taken place among jungle dwellers. Since World War II, however, in the wake of enormous affluence from the recently discovered offshore oil and gas deposits, the country has been undergoing an extraordinarily rapid social change. The villages, formerly accessible only by river boat and jungle tracking, are now visited frequently by helicopters that bring, among other things, sanitation, insect control, free medical services, and supplies. A network of new roads is rapidly invading the jungle and schools are springing up in nearly every neighborhood among formerly illiterate tribal people. Finally the state, in the person of the Sultan, is encouraging everyone to adopt the religion of Islam. In the face of these multifaceted social pressures, the rural people have adapted remarkably well, at the same time holding tenaciously to their extremely cohesive family structure and their traditional animistic religious beliefs that go back thousands of years.

Our work was made possible by our association with two people, on the scene, Barbara Harrisson, an anthropologist and John Moran, a physician with the British Army assigned to the Royal Brunei Malay Regiment. Both had spent more than a dozen years in Brunei in contact with the rural jungle tribes. They knew the territory, the people, and spoke their language. They shepherded us throughout our visit. We went by foot, by boat and by helicopter and were able to visit twelve of the villages, mainly long houses of the Iban tribe, erstwhile head hunters who have given up the practice.

It was evident that despite recent rapid social change there prevailed at the time, an essentially healthy state among the inhabitants of the villages of rural Borneo. People were living to very old age. Dr. Moran told us that in thirteen years of examining and treating the rural tribal people he had never seen a myocardial infarction or a stroke. Similarly, from our examinations, we found no evidence of systemic hypertension, myocardial infarction, rheumatoid arthritis, peptic ulcer, or ulcerative colitis. Figures 3.1 and 3.2 show mortality, population and epidemiological data. Tentative conclusions from this brief study are suggested by our previous experience with the Italian community of Roseto, Pennsylvania, whose salubrious state of health appears to have lasted only as long as old world attitudes and traditions were maintained while adapting to American economic and political patterns (Wolf et al., 1974). In order to test the implied social hypothesis, we ventured a prediction that, as the newly educated youth of rural Borneo grow up in a world alien to their unschooled parents, and as the anxiety relieving powers of old traditions and practices are eroded, the chronic diseases of western society may at last make their appearance. Maybe, maybe not. The answer must await an opportunity to make a return trip in a few years, the Sultan permitting. Either way, the results will be interesting and informative.

People Need People

Marshalling evidence concerning the relevance of psychological and social forces to health and disease involves taking into account identifiable but nonquantifiable aspects of human interaction, a process that anthropologists and other social scientists are comfortable with but which is foreign to most of us whose background is in physical sciences and biology. Since the forces involved in sociobiological phenomena cannot be weighed or precisely measured, one must have recourse to the perceptive and descriptive skills of the investigator. No available hardware can do this job. The human computer is required, a far more complex and sophisticated instrument than the largest electronic device but, interestingly, the product of volunteer labor.

While social attitudes and values and such emotions as anxiety, fear, and feelings of abandonment on the one hand and, on the other, love, loyalty, and trust cannot be quantified, they are relatively easily identified and certainly must not be dropped from consideration. There is very persuasive evidence that the lack of human warmth can have a disastrously stunting effect on the growth and development of infants (Dennis, 1957). The mortality rate among infants cared for without adequate direct human contact and reassurance is alarmingly high despite good sanitation and adequate food. Even among adults the sudden loss of love, especially with the death of a spouse, may increase the risk of death,

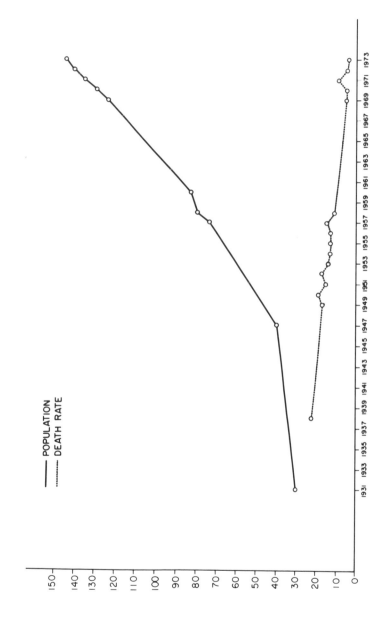

Figure 3.1
Rapidly Rising Population in Brunei Associated with a Sharp Decline in Death Rate

Figure 3.2
Precipitous Decline in Infectious Diseases Following the
Installation of Public Health Measures

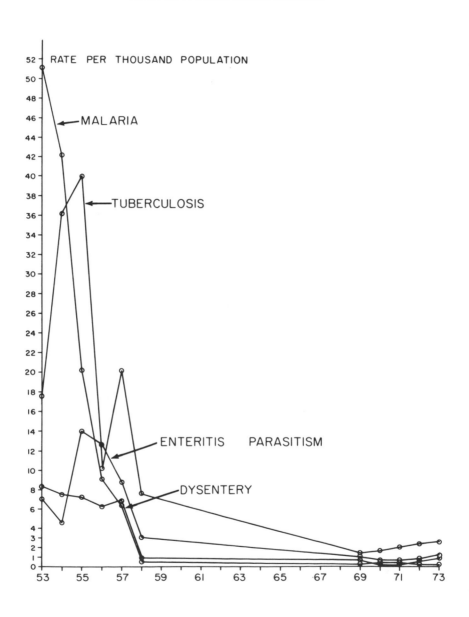

especially sudden death. Other epidemiological data clearly relate recent bereavement to a predisposition to sudden death. (Parkes, 1967; Rees and Lutkins, 1967). Lynch has learned from published reports that the death rate from heart disease is two to five times higher among those who are single, widowed, or divorced than among married people (Lynch, 1977). He calls particular attention to the contrasting statistics in two neighboring states, Nevada and Utah. While they have about the same population and roughly the same ethnic mix, Nevada, marked by fragile and fracturing human relationships, has one of the highest mortality rates from myocardial infarction of any state of the union. In contrast its neighbor, Utah, where family ties are strong, traditions are well entrenched and divorce is uncommon, has one of the lowest. It is strange that such striking evidence has been largely ignored in the cardiovascular literature and in the material circulated to the public by the American Heart Association. Lynch suggests that the strategy of the war on heart disease should include a war on loneliness. He points out that although the recognition that human contact is a source of the spread of disease and death was a landmark discovery in medicine, it is also necessary to recognize that "human relationships" may function to prevent disease and death.

As loneliness, frustration, and self-doubts appear to have pathogenic significance, self-esteem, self-confidence, and optimism may be conducive to health. In any case, it seems appropriate to supplement our consideration of emotional stress with attention to forces that counteract stress and sustain the person. Among them may be numbered strong and confident religious beliefs, family solidarity, and all manner of love relationships as well as the satisfaction of achievement and a sense of purpose in activities.

Social and Personal Values

The importance of values to social as well as bodily health led to the emergence of the professions, religion, law, and medicine whose task it was to stabilize the social structure and to serve, guide, and protect the people from their own missteps and mishaps. Those of us in medicine may well heed the words of Roscoe Pound, former dean of the Harvard Law School. He spoke of the meaning of the word profession in his 1949 lecture to the Massachusetts Medical Society as follows:

When we speak of the old recognized professions...we mean an organized calling in which men pursue a learned art and are united in the pursuit of it as a public service—no less a public service because they make a livelihood thereby...gaining of a livelihood is not a professional consideration. Indeed, the professional spirit, the spirit of a public service, constantly curbs the urge of the instinct. (Pound, 1949)

In *The Decline and Fall of the Roman Empire* (1827) Edward Gibbon described a population whose citizens had become insensitive to their civil responsibilities, being more concerned with their livelihood than with contributing to their society. Referring to the Athenians he wrote that, "In the end more than they wanted freedom, they wanted security, they wanted a comfortable life and in their quest for it all, security, comfort, freedom they lost it all. When what Athenians wanted finally was not to give to society but for society to give to them; when the freedom they wished for most was the freedom from responsibility, then Athenians ceased to be free." To take responsibility for the care of the patient requires not only identifying the patient's problem but understanding the patient's needs or, as Mark Altschule put it, "listening to the patient's message" (Altschule, 1989).

The patient's message may convey not only symptoms but individual needs and vulnerabilities and in addition, as noted above, valuable clues to the solution of the medical problem. Learning how to listen to the patient's message and how to analyze and deal with its contents defines pretty well a major aim of medical education. It describes in essence the role of the "primary physician."

Notes

1. An erudite and absorbing documentation of this view is contained in the book, *Profession of Conscience: The Making and Meaning of Life-Sciences Liberalism* by Robert H. Sprinkle (Sprinkle, 1994).
2. Rudolf Virchow (1821–1902) was a member of the Prussian lower house and, after the unification of Germany, was elected to the Reichstag where he served from 1880 to 1893, vigorously opposing the policies of Bismarck.
3. In another publication Leo Simmons discusses a deeply ingrained belief of Hopi American Indians, that a sore ankle would result from stepping on a fresh track of rattlesnakes following their copulation. Fortunately the tribe's medicine men had available a reliable counter-magic potion that could eliminate the pain. By the time of Simmons' study the younger generation of Hopi did not take seriously the healing rites of the medicine men, but nevertheless got painful ankles after stepping on the track of a post-copulating pair of snakes, illustrating that, in a deteriorating culture, its anxiety producing factors outlasted the anxiety reducing antidotes (Simmons, 1950).

4

Research

Asking the Question

Sound progress in research depends upon the investigator's ability to ask meaningful and relevant questions of nature. Often to ask the right question requires a certain vantage point of science, one that affords a view beyond conventional limits. Thus, new points of view about man and his nature yield new questions about the basis of health and disease.

The history of science, having gone through successive stages of analysis and synthesis, has paralleled closely developments in philosophical thought. Conceptual approaches have been, at times, highly compartmentalized and at times global. The need to differentiate has repeatedly been succeeded by a need to unite. For example, physics, chemistry, and biology were differentiated earlier among the natural sciences as distinct disciplines, distinct in subject matter and method of study. In recent years there has been a need for synthesis, even among physical chemistry, biochemistry, biophysics, and the broadly comprehensive, yet specialized, field of molecular biology as well. Similarly, medical disciplines that were utterly distinct twenty-five years ago, such as oncology, allergy, virology, and genetics were brought into a startling unity by the discovery of DNA and RNA, and progress has been everywhere accelerated by an increasingly unified concept of disease.

Scientific inquiry begins with careful observation that may trigger an idea to be tested. The traditional requirement for testing the validity of an idea or hypothesis has been experimentation. As in the case of Archimedes or Newton, however, an observation may constitute in itself a discovery, but more often it leads to an inference or hypothesis about the relation of things in nature. The observer asks himself "What is the underlying principle here?" An experiment to test the hypothesis usually requires perturbing the system under study and measuring the change. Whether the experiment shows the hypothesis to be right or wrong, the result yielded becomes the next observation. As Claude Bernard has said, "There is no such thing as a completely negative experiment." This leads to the next question and the next experiment, and so on. Finally, when the study allows a conclusion, a law or principle may be formulated.

Some theories may be tested by methods other than experimentation. Astronomers and astrophysicists, who must work at a distance of millions of miles from their subjects, can only observe the behavior of the heavenly bodies repeatedly without actually modifying or manipulating them. Nevertheless, they are able to test the validity of their formulations by making predictions before observing the outcome. The clinical investigator may not only use the method of the astronomers but can also manipulate the setting or the stimuli acting on his subjects.

Integrating Available Data

Spurts in knowledge have occurred when discoveries made in several specialized areas were brought together as, for example, in the discovery of the structure of DNA. In a fashion similar to solving a jigsaw puzzle, Watson and Crick put together bits of evidence turned up by other investigators in physics, chemistry, and biology until the picture of DNA began to emerge.

The task required very little laboratory work on their part, but a great deal of thought and close attention to what others were doing. Frederick Griffith had laid the first stone for the immense edifice of molecular biology by his discovery in 1928 of the transforming factor[1] that sixteen years later Oswald Avery, Colin MacLeod, and Maclyn McCarty identified as DNA (Portugal & Cohen, 1977).

Borrowing their strategy from Linus Pauling, Watson and Crick worked with toy-like models of purine and pyrimidine bases and phosphorylated carbohydrates, tools that were very much like the pieces of a jigsaw puzzle. Their task of fitting the pieces together was greatly facilitated by a discovery by the physical chemist, Erwin Chargaff, that the number of adenine molecules in DNA equalled those of thymine, while the number of guanines equalled the cytosines. From the physicist Pasqual Jordan, they borrowed the discovery that the replication of genes involves attractive forces on a flat surface. Throughout their wrestling match with their models, clues from the x-ray diffraction work of Rosalind Franklin were of crucial importance, especially her evidence that the sugar-phosphate backbone was located on the outside rather than the inside of the DNA molecule. Finally, and ironically, their success was made possible by a chance meeting with John Griffith, a nephew of Frederick Griffith. From John, they learned that the attractive forces of adenine and thymine would cause them to stick to each other by their flat surfaces. The two puzzle solvers were then able to show that a proposed structure of DNA published by Pauling did not fit with the available facts, but, nevertheless, the lack of "fit" was highly instructive to them. Then, thanks to a paper by Jordan and Guillard, they learned that by fitting hydrogen bonds between the bases, they were able to complete the puzzle and establish the structure of DNA.

Watson and Crick succeeded in synthesizing the information available to them because they understood the languages of sister disciplines. Unfortunately today's pattern of federal support of research does not encourage young investigators to emphasize perspective and relatedness but rewards narrowly circumscribed approaches and thereby discourages synthesis. Indeed a research proposal describing what Watson and Crick planned to do would very likely not have been funded in this country. This is unfortunate because there is probably more knowledge available that is pertinent to our individual problems than we realize and certainly more than today's peer reviewers would be aware of. Although such knowledge may be sequestered in technically restricted "fields," it nevertheless awaits the perceptive mind capable of making a connection with information hidden away elsewhere. When linked together such pieces of a puzzle may begin to reveal an emerging pattern, recognition of which might suggest crucial experiments that could further accelerate progress. It is part of the responsibility of the serious investigator to cultivate perspective and to integrate seemingly disparate information. Otherwise they may produce just fragments of a solution.

The Quality of Evidence

"Fixity of purpose requires flexibility of method"
—H.G. Wolff, 1952

More than thirty years ago, in a paper called *Strong Inference*, J.R. Platt, a biophysicist at the University of Chicago, wrote a prescription for establishing dependable scientific evidence (Platt, 1964). It required identifying plausible alternate hypotheses and testing them against the conclusion being proposed. To mount such a challenge may require a shift away from an investigator's customary methods and techniques of approach, but thereby, the alternate hypothesis may be excluded, or, on the other hand, one of them may replace the original inference. As antecedent to such a strategy, Platt credited Francis Bacon's proposal, published in the early seventeenth century, of a branching method of reasoning that proceeded from alternative hypotheses (Bacon, 1960). He also cited the nineteenth-century geologist, T.C. Chamberlin, who developed further the method of multiple working hypotheses placed in competition with one another by experimental testing (Chamberlin, 1897). Today, statistical treatment of data is often substituted for an experimental challenge to an hypothesis. Concerning such sometimes false comfort derived from numbers, Platt wrote:

> Today we preach that science is not science unless it is quantitative. We substitute correlations for causal studies and physical equations for organic reasoning.... Measurements and equations...tend to become the object of scientific manipulation instead of auxiliary tests of crucial inferences.... Many, perhaps most, of the great issues of science are qualitative, not quantitative, even in physics and chemistry. Equations and measurements are useful when and only when they are related to proof...We measure, we define, we compute, we analyze, but we do not exclude. (Platt, 1964)

Walter Reed's search for the cause of yellow fever more than ninety years ago established a model for dealing with competing hypotheses in clinical investigation (Bean, 1982). The epidemiology of the disease strongly favored contagion, poor sanitation, or person-to-person contact, although there were some features that did not fit those speculations. Reed verified the mosquito vector hypothesis through experiments that tested all of the competing theories. His work vividly reinforced the lesson that we should rely on probability measures to suggest hypotheses and look to other methods of inquiry to test them.

The failure to exclude is well illustrated by the initial investigation of the dive reflex in ducks by Paul Bert that led him to conclude that the animal's ability to keep its head under water was due to its naturally high red blood cell count and hence its ability to store oxygen (Bert, 1879). Bert's pupil, Charles Richet, challenged his inference with experiments directed at alternate hypotheses (Richet, 1894). In the first experiment, based on Bert's hypothesis, he bled the ducks to reduce their red cell mass and found that depleting the red cell mass had no effect on the dive reflex. In a second experiment, Richet tied the tracheas of two groups of ducks, holding one group under water and leaving the other on land. The ducks with occluded tracheas left on land all died within six or seven minutes while those held under water survived an average of twenty-one minutes. Richet's experiments had thus excluded Bert's storage hypothesis and replaced it with a hypothesis of oxygen conservation through bradycardia triggered by face immersion, thus revealing the power of strong inference.

Not only in physics, but in biomedical research as well, measurement or quantification has become the sine qua non of medical science although a great many important discoveries have been made without the benefit of quantitative data. René Dubos, who was the first to discover the antibiotic properties of cultures of certain unicellular organisms (soil bacteria) deplored the growing imperative for mathematical analysis in the search for truth, complaining of circumstances in which: "the most measurable drives out the more important" (Dubos, 1959).

The nature of acceptable experimental evidence varies with what is being investigated and under what circumstances. For example, to discover whether or not concentrating the light of the sun through a magnifying glass will ignite a newspaper would require only one positive observation because there are no possible alternative inferences. Hence, there would be no need to repeat the process several times. As a case in point, Claude Bernard, in his *Introduction to Experimental Medicine*, described the experience of:

> making an animal artificially diabetic by means of a puncture in the floor of the fourth ventricle. But I afterwards had the experience of repeating the experiment many times (eight or ten times) without getting the same results. Let me assume that, instead of succeeding at once in making a rabbit diabetic, all the negative facts had first appeared; it is clear that, after failing two or three times, I should have concluded not only that the theory guiding me was false, but that puncture of the fourth ventricle did not produce diabetes. Yet I should have been wrong. How often men must have been and still must be wrong in this way! So an experimenter can never deny a fact that he has seen and observed, merely because he cannot rediscover it. (Bernard, 1926)

Bernard's important discovery of the involvement of the central nervous system in glucose metabolism would be called anecdotal today as is most descriptive evidence, and is thereby scorned. A similar example was Bernardo Houssay's discovery of the involvement of the anterior pituitary in the mechanism of diabetes (Houssay, 1967). His report, re-peatedly rejected by important medical journals, eventually won him the Nobel Prize in 1947.

The Role of Statistics

Used as preliminary test of an hypothesis, statistics can be very help-ful, especially in establishing a null hypothesis. On the other hand, a high correlation can be very misleading.

During a scarcity of Japanese silk, the Du Pont company developed, and soon began to market nylon stockings. Shortly thereafter the tobacco companies were donating huge quantities of cigarettes to American troops involved in World War II. An absurd, but striking correlation occurred. Both the rising numbers of cigarette smokers and the increase in sales of nylon stockings closely paralleled the prevalence of cancer of the lung from 1938 to 1950. thus, statistics provide the probability of an associa-tion but do not establish a cause. Alternate plausible hypotheses must be sought and pursued. Nevertheless, such rules of evidence are often ig-nored. Correlations based on large numbers of cases, but without ad-equate attention to possible biasing factors, are often reported at national meetings or in journals, even without a prior hypothesis. When offered to the media, as they often are, they may be broadcast to the nation as recent medical discoveries.

One of the most fatuous was spread across the nation on Veteran's Day in 1991. The announcement on television and in newspapers quoted a finding presented at the annual meeting of the American Heart Asso-ciation informing the world that short men are more susceptible than tall men to myocardial infarction (Hebert et al., 1991). The study had been carried out only on male physicians aged forty to eighty-four who were followed for eight years. The six authors of the report speculated that a presumably smaller caliber of coronary arteries of the shorter physicians may have been a risk factor. At best correlative techniques can establish a probability of association but not cause. The very impersonal nature of the epidemiological method, with its reliance on standard criteria and relatively large numbers, tends to blur characteristics of individuals, groups, or cultures that may be significant, thereby robbing the shrewd and perceptive investigator of his opportunity to detect subtleties that may be important. In the intensely competitive environment of today's research, it is dangerous for investigators to be so sharply focused on their own line of thought that they are unaware of alternate hypotheses or, out of pride of ownership, may resist or even oppose them.

Replication as Evidence

Replicability and verifiability by others are generally required elements of acceptable evidence, but when certain conditions that may affect the outcome of an experiment are unknown or ignored, attempts at replication may be misleading. A vivid example is the replicability of the dive reflex already mentioned. It is a phylogenetically ancient cardiovascular-metabolic pattern that protects an organism against hypoxia during breath-hold diving. Although human beings display all the elements of the reflex (bradycardia, vasoconstriction in skin, muscles, and viscera, and reduced tissue metabolism) when the face is immersed in water the reflex may be exaggerated or completely inhibited, depending on the emotional and cognitive state of the subject. We ascertained some years ago that the reflex responses are exaggerated when the subject is frightened and becomes totally inhibited when the subject is concentrating or preoccupied with outside concerns (Wolf, 1964). Thus, attempts at verification by other investigators might fail because of their neglect of potentially confounding subtle prevailing circumstances. Such qualifiers of the consistency of the dive reflex are not only operative in conscious humans, but in dogs and seals as well (Wolf, 1967). These and other examples teach us that many bodily adjustments are nonlinear. That is that results depend, not only on the stimulus itself, but on incidental outside influences that may perturb the adaptive system. Predictions, therefore, must be made with knowledge of all prevailing conditions and contingencies. In testing groups of subjects, statistics will not provide predictive information on individuals who may differ from one another in their ways of responding.

Although statistical studies afford a valuable means of classifying groups of individuals, they do not contribute to the understanding of individual patients so essential in clinical practice. What can be learned from observation and dialogue, once the source of important clues, has been devalued by clinical researchers. Even teaching at the bedside has been nearly abandoned, as Mark D. Altschule reminded us in his book *Essays on the Rise and Decline of Bedside Medicine* (Altschule, 1989).[2]

Today, therefore, without a great deal of attention to the person, most investigations that involve human subjects are essentially correlative, that is, epidemiological studies validated by statistics. Patients are considered in groups assumed to be more less homogeneous. In some ways they may be. For example, Harold Wolff and associates showed that in healthy subjects there is a more or less uniform sensory threshold for pain, but his studies also found that there is no uniformity from person to person with respect to emotional, visceral, or somatic responses to pain (Wolff, 1940, 1943). Thus, while the stimulus and the response are objective and quantifiable, there is not a linear relationship between the two. The responses to pain are shaped by the intangible meaning of the painful experience to the individual. Thus, as sensory receptors transmit life experience to the evaluative circuitry of the brain, unique to each of us, our responses are not necessarily predictable from the nature of the sensory signals. They may vary from person to person and from time to time in the same person. While the neurons and neurotransmitters that do the work of interpreting sensations are standard items of equipment, the product of their excitatory and inhibitory interactions is anything but standard. Measuring a stimulus does not objectify its message.

The Need for Relevance to the Individual Under Study

During the long period when investigators thought of the brain as an impregnable black box, many sought to objectify their experiments on effects of psychological and social forces on the body through a uniform, presumably stressful stimulus. Mental arithmetic became a relatively stable favorite despite the fact that mental arithmetic, though onerous or even frightening to some, is fun for others. Since more has been learned of the central pathways that make our assessments, more attention has been paid to readily discernable but intangible qualities of a subject, his or her proclivity for caution or risk, for example. Serious attention to intangibles is as important in science as it is in life. Subtle indications of habitual honesty, generosity, conscientiousness, and dependability are what we use to make some of the most important judgments of our lives. As seductive as numbers may seem as a basis for judgment, unless they accurately describe the objective being sought, they may, like grade point averages, or the weight of a candidate's reprints, or even some statistical manipulations, betray the truth.

Marshalling the Evidence

The kind of evidence usually required to verify an observation or discovery includes replication by another investigation in another institution or, perhaps, by several other investigators. The rules also demand that measurements be repeatable to verify that the changes observed are not random but are statistically significant.

In the initial investigation of a physiologic or biochemical finding, quantifiable and replicable data may be obtained when the observed phenomenon is isolated from extraneous influences. For example, the electrophysiologist may devise ways to screen out or compensate for background "noise" in order to verify data recorded from various dynamic bodily systems. Such strategies may risk error, however, when what were presumed to be extraneous influences were actually highly relevant recorded data. Thus, what is taken for noise may reflect unrecognized influences of associated events stemming from the person's interpretation of the stimulus. Thereby is documented the nonlinearity of the process. Hence, although one can measure and record physiologic and biochemical responses with remarkable precision, one cannot achieve comparable measurements of a person's interpretation or internal processing of the significance of an event. Thus, verification by other investigators or by repeated documentation of observed change may not be possible with respect to the impact of psychosocial forces on people, because a life experience can hardly be precisely replicated in all its manifestations and meanings. Moreover, the human organism itself is rarely to be found in an identical state of response on two occasions separated by the passage of time and the impact of other events. Thus, a blind preoccupation with quantification, replication, and the elimination of observer bias may serve to obscure important data including the intangible idiosyncratic meaning of an experience to the affected individual.

Science and the Intangible

To observe (L. *servare* in Latin) is to pay heed to what is before you (L.). Straying a bit from its Latin root, "thrown toward or over against," the term *objective*, refers to "anything that is visible or tangible."

Subjective, (thrown under) has come to mean "existing in the mind." We experience the tangible through visual, auditory, olfactory, gustatory, thermal, tactile, and other internal and external receptors. Such sensory signals are more or less quantifiable but their message must be appreciated by the mind through the vastly complex evaluative circuitry of the brain.

Interpersonal Influences

The methods and approaches of anthropology allow for highly systematic and thorough studies of people behaving in their normal environment. Such studies could also include measurements of bodily functions by modern, highly sophisticated technical devices. Anthropologists and others who study social configurations are concerned with the effects attributable to the influence of individuals on one another. In medicine, this is recognized most typically in the salubrious effect that the presence of a concerned physician may have on his patient. Horsley Gantt, who made extensive studies of this, called it the "effect of person" (Gantt, 1972). He quoted an observation of Charles Darwin describing the effect the presence of his physician father had on a patient with an irregular heartbeat which "invariably became regular as soon as my father entered the room."

This useful aspect of medical practice is less evident today as modern doctors vary widely in their capacity to relieve suffering by their presence. The clinical significance of the effect of person has been explored by James Lynch, who was able to show that loneliness and lack of human companionship contributed significantly to the hazard of fatal cardiac arrhythmia or myocardial infarction (Lynch, 1977). On the other hand, he found that strengthening human relationships and fulfillment of emotional needs were important to the avoidance of heart disease. Lynch's work emphasizes the importance to the physician of understanding his patient and the way the patient interprets and responds to troublesome life events (Rahe, 1978).

Nonlinear Dynamics (Chaos Theory)

The unpredictability of response to a clear-cut stimulus, so characteristic of physiological adaptations of highly integrated human subjects, has been profitably studied by applying the approach of chaos theory to biology. The mathematics of chaos was originally resorted to in the study of inanimate materials such as winds and weather, turbulence of water, and the movements of gas molecules, protons, and so on. The idea that such phenomena could be understood and their outcome predicted, if the number of influencing factors (dimensions) were small enough to calculate, came from the work of Henri Poincaré (1854–1912). On the other hand, when the influencing forces are too numerous to calculate, he found that the outcome cannot be precisely predicted so the process must then be considered random. Randomness, however, does not imply that a process is not deterministic but merely that the variables are too numerous to allow for calculation by modern computer technology.

However obvious it appears from what has been said that the adaptive behavior of complex organisms is clearly nonlinear and hence should be approachable by the techniques of chaos theory, its actual application to physiological data has been hampered by serious difficulties such as the very instability of adaptive behavior referred to as the problem of nonstationarity. Important progress in overcoming this difficulty has been achieved by Skinner and colleagues with the development of the point correlation dimension (PD2i) (Skinner et al., 1993).

Volume 29, Number 3 (July–September, 1994) of the journal *Integrative Physiological and Behavioral Science* surveys the evidence relating chaos to physiology, especially with respect to the brain and heart. It contains articles from an impressive list of scientists from Brussels, Belgium; Constance, Muenster, and Tübingen in Germany; Budapest in Hungary; Ramat-Gan in Israel; and California, Georgia, Illinois, Massachusetts, New Mexico, Oregon, Pennsylvania, Texas, Virginia and Washington, D.C. in the United States.

Although several important books on chaos theory have appeared in the last few years, it is striking that the basic ideas for dealing with complex interactive systems that regulate adaptive processes in human physiology, were not first introduced by medical neuroscientists, biochemists, or physiologists, but by physicists.

Clinical Research

The idea that a patient's nature has a good deal to do with the nature of his or her illness is an old one. From time to time, however, it has been difficulty to fit the concept into prevailing philosophical thinking. For example, the views of Pierre Gassendi (1592–1655) and of John Locke

(1632–1704) were far more hospitable to the idea of the unity of mind and body than were those of René Descartes (1596–1650), who believed that mental and emotional functions were entirely separate from muscular and visceral activities (Descartes, 1668). Gassendi and Locke, on the other hand, believed that all mental and emotional activities, as well as bodily behaviors, are generated in response to sensory information from one's surroundings (Gassendi, 1971; Dewhurst, 1963). A century later their ideas were institutionalized by Etienne Bonnot de Condillac (1715–1780), one of a group of "idealogues" who gathered at the salon of Madame Helvetius in Paris (Kennedy, 1979) to discuss the problems of the world and the nature of man. Their fellow member, Pierre Jean George Cabanis (1757–1808), further evolved a unified concept of the mind-body relationship based on physiology. In 1796 he proposed that thoughts and emotions, as well as general somatic and visceral behavior, are shaped, not only by new experiences perceived through the senses and freshly processed in the brain, but also by remote and long-forgotten experiences stored somehow in the brain (Cabanis, 1981). Thus, he came close to the notion of the unconscious. Cabanis also suggested that differences in thoughts and behavior must, in part, reflect distinctive features of each human brain, adding that "according to one's state of mind and according to the different nature of the ideas and the moral affections, the activity of the organs can by turns be stimulated, suspended, or entirely reversed (Cabanis, 1981, p. 650).

The teachings of the idealogues were popular among medical students in nineteenth-century France, among them Charles Richet, who was to become professor of physiology at the University of Paris. Richet, who was interested in psychology, considered it to be part of physiology (Richet, 1885). In the United States, Walter B. Cannon, who held similar views, was in close touch with developments in Europe. He knew Charles Richet, and, in fact, in a Festschrift for Richet in 1926, Cannon reported on the preliminary work that led to his famous concept of homeostasis (Cannon, 1926). Three years later (1929–1930) Cannon was in Paris again, serving as exchange professor from Harvard.

By the late 1930s and thereafter, thanks to the influence of Walter Cannon's work and the teachings of Adolph Meyer, the professor of psychiatry at Johns Hopkins University, the experimental study of mind-body relationships in human subjects had begun to attract an interdisciplinary range of medical scientists. Among them were Stanley

Cobb, Soma Weiss, and their colleagues in Boston, Harold Wolff and his group in New York; Eugene Ferris and his associates in Cincinnati; Edward Weiss and his colleagues in Philadelphia; Robert Livingston at Yale; George Saslow in St. Louis; Roy Grinker in Chicago; J.J. Groen in Jerusalem; and Alberto Zanchetti and his group in Milan. Others experimented with animals, including Horsley Gantt and Curt Richter in Baltimore; Howard Liddell and his group in Ithaca, New York; David Rioch and his research department at Walter Reed Hospital in Washington; and Hans Selye in Montreal.

Many of these workers and several others from the United States and Canada participated in establishing in 1943 the American Society for Research in Psychosomatic Problems. Shortly before that Mrs. Kate Macy Ladd, who in 1936 had founded the Josiah Macy, Jr. Foundation, directed the foundation to provide support for the fledgling field of psychosomatic investigation. The foundation first financed the remarkable bibliographic and editorial work of Helen Flanders Dunbar at Columbia's College of Physicians and Surgeons in New York and later assisted in founding the journal *Psychosomatic Medicine*, which first appeared in 1939. The membership of the society during the early years included an impressive array of psychiatrists, physiologists, endocrinologists, neurologists, psychologists, internists, and representatives of several medical subspecialties, all of whom were intent on exploring the relationships of life experiences to health and disease. Walter Cannon was a member of the society, as was Adolph Meyer, who after presiding at the first meeting, continued as honorary president. In 1948 the society was renamed the American Psychosomatic Society.

In 1946 the Commonwealth Fund established at the University of Cincinnati and at Cornell-New York Hospital in New York City educational programs designed to teach young internists sufficient psychology and psychiatry to enable them to deal effectively with the social and emotional aspects of illness and thereby to influence medical education. At Cornell we sought to equip our Commonwealth Fund fellows for posts in academic medicine. Their curriculum consisted of spending each morning in an outpatient clinic taking care of patients under supervision and each afternoon in the laboratory, using their clinic patients as subjects for research into the disease that affected them. The purpose of the research was, of course, pedagogical as well as to generate new knowledge on the relevance of psychological and social forces to the pathophysiologic changes involved in symptoms and disease. In part, however, the purpose was therapeutic, to understand the patient and his disturbed physiology in order to help him or her to comprehend the psychological and social forces at work and cope with them. We often used the stress interview to elicit physiological and chemical responses. Topics for discussion were selected from what had been learned from careful study of the patient in the clinic. Thus, the stress applied was not only relevant to the patient, in contrast to so-called standard stresses such as mental arithmetic and horror movies, but it was able to provide therapeutic leverage as well. George Engel emphasized in his essay in *The Task of Medicine*, reviewed in the Winter 1990 issue of *The Pharos*, that "dialogue is truly foundational to scientific work in the clinical realm" (Engel, 1988).

By 1950 enough significant research had been done to fill the huge volume *Life Stress and Bodily Disease*, which was published as the proceedings of the Association for Research in Nervous and Mental Diseases (Wolff et al., 1950). Thirty years later a reprise by the association mangaged a volume only one-third in size, although in the interim, major technical advances had made it possible to record chemical and physiological responses of human subjects with greater ease and remarkable accuracy (Weiner et al., 1981).

The Decline of Human Experimentation

The first research ward in the United States where patient volunteers were the subjects of research was established in 1910 at the Rockefeller Institute in New York City. John D. Rockefeller, Sr. made it very clear in his gift that the research was to be directed at curing or alleviating prevalent diseases. Many brilliant clinically relevant discoveries emerged from the Rockefeller hospital where patient-subjects might remain for periods from a month to more than a year. Soon other institutions, Harvard, Cornell, and Hopkins established their own research wards and later on the NIH itself established an intramural clinical research facility. After that, for a few years, the NIH supported clinical research centers at several medical schools.

In the late 1960s, when the emphasis in medical research began to take a more reductionistic direction toward molecular biology and genetics, patient-oriented research at the Rockefeller hospital was curtailed in favor of pure laboratory research. Other institutions soon followed suit.

The decline in what he called patient-oriented research is vividly described in Edward Ahrens' book, *The Crisis in Clinical Research* (Ahrens, 1992).

As the study of human biology had begun to incorporate more and more the concepts and methods of physics and mathematics, there developed an increasingly urgent demand for quantitative measurement and statistical testing in all investigations. Reports of careful observational studies of individuals were often scorned as anecdotal and either abandoned by their proposers or modified in a procrustean way to fit a contrived system of measurement or scoring. Interest in experimental studies of individual human subjects in the tradition of William Beaumont's classical work with his fistulous subject Alexis St. Martin had been all but abandoned by the mid 1960s, (Beaumont, 1833) giving way to epidemiological surveys, psychological testing, often coupled with measurements of hormones and neurotransmitters in the general circulation, and other techniques that did not require extended dialogue with the subject or close attention to the patient as a person.

On the other hand, significant afferent information may be shut out entirely if psychological forces are ignored. Hernandez-Peon's classical experiment in which he recorded electrical action potentials from the cochlear nucleus of the cat produced by the ticking of a metronome clearly illustrates the force of an emotionally significant event. When a mouse was brought into the cat's line of vision, the action potentials ceased while the metronome continued ticking (Hernandez-Peon et al., 1956). Other sensory and motor functions may be inhibited by concentration on or distraction to another focus of attention. As an example, unregulated influences from wayward circuits in the basal ganglia such as the tremor in Parkinson's syndrome may be inhibited by concentration on a manual task. While playing music, or even imagining they are playing music, musicians affected with the syndrome of Giles de la Tourette have experienced complete loss of their symptoms (Sacks, 1990). Pharmacologic stimuli, too, may also be turned off or distorted. We were able to eliminate nausea with a dose of the emetic ipecac delivered through a stomach tube when the subject believed she was being given an anti-nausea drug and we were able to induce nausea by water in the same subject when she thought she was receiving ipecac (Wolf, 1950). Further, by will or hypnosis, one can change not only what is felt but what happens in tissues as well. Bilisoly, Goodell, and Wolff (1954) were able, by hypnotic suggestions of anesthesia, to limit blister formation on one arm from heat applied to the skin. At the same time, they enhanced blister formation on the other arm by suggesting during hypnosis that the skin was sore and highly vulnerable (Bilisoly et al., 1954).

In view of these findings, familiar to many, it is clear that in human experimentation, meticulously recorded data derived from seemingly identical experimental procedures may vary from person to person and from time to time in the same individual. Since it is the intrusion of contingencies between stimulus and response that fashion the variety of physiological reactions to presumably standardized stimuli, replicability cannot necessarily be viewed as the required criterion of reliability.

The futility of expecting uniform responses from individuals exposed to identical stimuli could be illustrated by reference to the behavior of a man having been suddenly struck in the face by the glove of another. His reaction to this readily quantifiable and standardizable stimulus is problematic. If the incident had occurred in seventeenth-century France the response would be quite predictable. The one struck would simply produce a visiting card as a challenge to a duel. In twentieth-century America, he might not even have a visiting card in his pocket. If he did, he would certainly not use it in this situation. His response would depend on a variety of contingencies, including whether or not he was bigger and stronger than the other fellow. The most important determinant, however, would be the character of his relationship with the chap who struck him. Depending on that and other factors, the man struck might fight back, might develop diarrhea or tachycardia, might faint with bradycardia, or might simply laugh and make a joke of the whole thing. This homely example illustrates how fruitless it would be to expect a uniform response from people, no matter how precisely one standardizes the psychological or social stimulus.

The Power of Observation

Experiments are not the only route to important discovery as Darwin's observations show. Revolutionary scientific progress has resulted from his astute descriptions and analyses of relationships in nature (Darwin, 1859). The discovery of imprinting in geese by Konrad Lorenz provides a more recent example of the potentially definitive nature of observation (Lorenz, 1965).

Darwin and Lorenz were natural scientists rather than experimental scientists. Their work could not possibly obey the rules often laid down for experimentalists: that "purely descriptive" findings lack validity and, for the findings to be fully acceptable, the observer should be "blind." The natural scientist relies heavily on his clarity of vision and his powers of observation as well as descriptive skills to gather and record his evidence. Intuition, a quality that includes the ability to recognize relationships and similarities that may elude the less sensitive observer and to see more in an ordinary event than a neighboring observer can see, is a powerful tool of the natural scientist who would be helpless if "blinded." So often would be the experimenter. William Beaumont, relying mainly on his own ingenuity and perspicacity, showed us the power of careful, systematic observation.[3] With very few tools he made a lasting contribution to our understanding of human physiology. In addition to what he was able to identify in St. Martin's stomach, his observations led him to assume the presence of a digestive substance beyond HCl, later discovered and identified as the enzyme pepsin (Beaumont, 1833).

The Experiment of Nature

In laboratory experiments one makes measurements before and after creating a deliberate perturbation of a biological system. To observe an experiment of nature requires no interference. One measures changes induced in the course of the subject's own life experience. Data from experiments of nature are especially powerful if one can make measurements prospectively over time and during evolving biological change. So it was with respect to the discovery of the power of measurements of heartbeat variability (sinus arrhythmia) as recorded from the R waves of the electrocardiogram to predict the likelihood of sudden arrhythmic death. The discovery that reduced variability of the R-R of the electrocardiogram is predictive of sudden arrhythmic death was made during a ten-year prospective study begun in 1960 of seventy-nine patients, fifty-nine men and twenty women aged thirty-six to seventy-six who had suffered a well documented myocardial infarction at sometime in the past (Wolf, 1995). The patients were individually matched with healthy controls for age, sex, race, height, weight, educational background, and type of job. Both patients and controls were reexamined and retested at intervals of six to eight weeks throughout the first seven years of the study.

Fifty-three patients died, seven of noncardiac disorders, two died of suicide. Forty-four, thirty-one men and thirteen women died suddenly of apparent MI. Thirty-one, or seventy percent of them, were autopsied. Eleven were found to have experienced a recent MI and twenty had only an old scar.

The average age of those who died was fifty-six and of survivors fifty-three. Age was not a determinant of cardiac mortality. Neither was the level of serum cholesterol concentration, the LDL/HDL ratio, or the treadmill test a significant determinant of death. The measured physiological data that did significantly correlate with the cardiac deaths at the 0.01 level of confidence were low RR variability or wide mean RR variation month to month.

Most such discoveries are preceded by important, fundamental observations by other scientists. With respect to RR variability, Wiersma, in 1913, from careful measurements of oscillations in heart rate, published convincing evidence that RR variability was under control of the forebrain (Wiersma, 1913). His careful study, carried out on a wide range of human subjects including anencephalic babies, adults with extensive brain damage, normal and depressed patients, was largely ignored. Later, Wenckebach (Wenckebach & Winterberg, 1927) and his pupil Scherf (Scherf & Bond, 1946) observed that low amplitude of RR variability in humans was associated with heart disease. In further studies of the effects of lesions in the brain on cardiac function, Valbona et al. found that the normally variable RR intervals became completely regular following various forebrain lesions and following decerebration that left only the pons and medulla intact. He and his colleagues also found totally uniform RR oscillations during deep anesthesia or coma. They also commented that their patients with neurological disorders who lacked RR variability invariably suffered a fatal outcome (Valbona, et al., 1965).

After the first six years of our study, the predictive significance of the RR was already evident. A manuscript submitted by Robert Schneider and Paul Costiloe, two of the collaborators in the study, made the observation that diminished RR variability was predictive of the risk of sudden death in the patients with coronary heart disease. Their paper was rejected for publication as "not of sufficient medical or physiological significance." Today virtually every cardiologist relies on reduced RR variability as a predictor of sudden death.[4]

Strong Inference

Often the most powerful and productive evidence comes from a clear and undeniable inference in the absence of concrete tangible support. Such inspired research has been credited to "the eye of the mind" as distinct from "the eye of the face." Galileo's inference concerning the rate of acceleration of falling bodies, even though he could not eliminate the influence of air resistance and currents, is a case in point, so is William Harvey's inference concerning the circulation of the blood when he was unable to demonstrate the capillary bridge between artery and vein. Harvey invoked a useful fiction for the path from arteries to veins. He assumed the existence of capillaries which could not be demonstrated until the later invention of the microscope. Such useful fictions that emerged from brilliant intuitions were provocatively discussed by Hans Vaihinger (1949) who noted that useful fictions, whether true or not, are often indispensable to the understanding of the relationship of things in nature. The concept of infinity is such a useful fiction. There is no way of proving it or of really grasping it, but mathematical research is heavily dependent on that fiction. The observations of Charles Darwin, which, if offered for the first time today, might be dismissed as anecdotal. His imaginative inferences from very acute and systematic observations yielded work, the influence of which on the development of biological science has hardly been equalled (Darwin, 1859). Darwin would probably be criticized today because his methods did not protect against the possibility of observer bias. Bias does, of course, muddy the waters; it should be avoided insofar as possible but not at the cost of sacrificing intuition and the capacity to make perceptive judgments. These provide the gateway to creative discovery.

Early Insights

The eighteenth-century physiologist, Cabanis, noted the visceral responses of individual subjects in a variety of emotional states. Anticipating Walter Cannon's later observations of inhibition of gastric secretion and motor activity in his frightened cats (Cannon, 1929), Cabanis wrote, "A vigorous and healthy man has just eaten a good meal; in the midst of this feeling of well-being, the foods that are at the moment carried to the various parts of the organism are energetically digested and the digestive juices dissolve them easily and quickly. Should this man receive bad news, or should sad and baneful passions suddenly arise in his soul, his stomach and intestines will immediately cease to act on the foods contained in them" (Cabanis, 1981, p. 650).

Cabanis also anticipated the findings of other investigators who observed acceleration and intensification of gastric functions in the face of situations that arouse aggressive emotions (Gordon & Chernya, 1940; Wolf & Wolff, 1947). Cabanis wrote, "Fear destroys and can annihilate the muscular forces. Joy, hope, courageous sentiments can multiply their effects tenfold; anger can increase them almost indefinitely" (Cabanis, 1981, p. 651).

Cabanis ideas, as bright and persuasive as they were, certainly did not carry the day or even the century. The late eighteenth century in Europe was a time of ceaseless debate over the mind-body issue, a debate that generated intense heat but little light. Nearly a century later, however, the remarkable insights into hysteria and other neurological disturbances achieved by Jean Louis Martin Charcot at the Salpetrière Clinic in Paris relied heavily on getting to know the patient as an individual. Ivan Pavlov, whose studies in St. Petersburg were taking place at the same time, viewed his dogs as individuals and thereby was able to show how specific canine characteristics were associated with differing responses to conditioning.

In these and other fruitful investigations, quantification, while always desirable, was not always applicable to the material under study, except in the measurement of functions at the end organ, which modern technology can achieve with such elegance. Nevertheless, the studies had a seminal influence on the progress of medical science. Thus, while always striving for quantification, replication, and elimination of bias, keen observation, and cogent inference must be central to the inquiry. With a deep respect for evidence and a balanced approach, modern technology can help to revive and enhance studies of the relevance of life experience to disease in experimental investigations using individual human beings. In fact, most advances in experimental medicine ultimately involve the participation of human subjects but not necessarily of patients. Most treatises that deal with problems of experimentation on humans were written in the 1940s and 1950s. Among them are those of Cochran (1955), Witts (1955), Shimkin (1953), Ivy (1948) and others.

Establishing Validity

Irrespective of the topic explored, the essential requirement of scientific inquiry is for valid, not necessarily tangible or quantifiable evidence. Validity is achieved by challenging an hypothesis, not merely by measuring its probability. Validity can also be established by predictability, as in astronomy and other aspects of physics. Prediction may be used to good effect in prospective research on the effects of stress. Here data on intangibles, such as various identifiable aspects of the personality and behavior of individuals or the characteristics of their social environment may be used as predictors.

A great deal of value has been learned from psychological testing, but a rigid protocol that excludes direct contact between investigator and subject sacrifices one of the scientist's most precious resources, direct observation of the subject's behavior.

Efforts to eliminate subjective bias by distancing the principal investigator from the subject, or attempting to achieve replicability by the use of standard forms and questionnaires administered by surrogates, may actually obscure important data. A powerful experimental method designed to reawaken in a subject the recollections and feelings associated with a past stressful experience is the stress interview. This technique, originated by Mittleman and Wolff (1942) in patients with peptic ulcer was further developed and applied to elicit a wide variety of measurable visceral responses. During 285 stress interviews carried out between 1941 and 1996, 86 percent of the sought-for observable psychological disturbances were elicited.

The Stress Interview

A requirement for effective use of the stress interview is first to have knowledge of the circumstances that have been associated with the symptoms in question. Next, a dialogue between subject and experimenter is required so that confidence is esatblished, as well as confidentiality, so that the subject feels adequately protected and willing to discuss his or her personal history during the recording of data.

The interview itself begins with a short baseline at rest followed by a "control period" characterized by a discussion of a pleasant topic for about fifteen minutes. Then the suspected topic of conflict is quietly introduced, with the interviewer speaking as little as possible for a period, and maintaining a neutral and slightly skeptical attitude, the length of which is set by the nature of the topic being discussed. At the end of the "stress" period the interviewer becomes understanding and supportive and switches the topic to a neutral subject. At the conclusion, following a brief period of rest and quiet, the interviewer speaks privately with the subject, explaining the procedure, encouraging and replying openly to questions. At the end of the explanation session or at a later time, most patients who have been subjects have expressed satisfaction and gratitude for what they have learned about their reactions. In fact the stress interview has often performed a salutary therapeutic function.

The stress interview takes advantage of the relevance of the life experience and emotional makeup of each individual subject, because the topic for discussion is selected from a circumstance that had been associated in time with his or her symptom or bodily disturbance under study (Wolf et al., 1948; Wolf, 1965; Wolf, 1966; Wolf, 1970; Wolf, 1985; Huang et al., 1989).

The Experimenter as a Research Subject

In many important studies the experimenter himself was the subject, as in the classical work of Blackley in 1873 who, by inducing the condition in himself and others, showed that hay fever was due to pollen circulating in the air (Witt, 1955). Almost a hundred years before, Purkinje had demonstrated the clinical picture of digitalis intoxication by giving himself a large overdose of the drug (Hanzlik, 1925). Another early experimenter who used himself as the subject was John R. Young. In 1803 he published the results of experiments in which he vomited recently swallowed food so that he could study the action of gastric juice (Young, 1803). There have been a great many experiments of this type. Some of them were hazardous. For example, from the studies of Halsted and associates on the local anesthetic effects of cocaine (Finney, 1940) serious addiction resulted. When some years later, Goldberger's experiments on the nature of pellagra were not meeting with acceptance among his colleagues, he undertook the heroic expedient of having himself, his wife, and four friends injected with blood from pellagrins to demonstrate that the disease was not infectious (Parsons, 1943). We now know that his experimental subjects were in no danger of contracting pellagra, but they might have succumbed to an incidental infection with homologous serum hepatitis. John Hunter in 1767 (Bett, 1954) showed even greater personal abandon when he inoculated himself with material from a patient who was suffering from gonorrhea, hoping to prove that gonorrhea and syphilis were separate diseases. His plan failed because the donor, unfortunately, was suffering from both diseases. Later in 1838, Record repeated Hunter's experiment and successfully demonstrated the separate identity of the two (Bett, 1954).

Some of the experiments that investigators have performed upon themselves seem to have been downright foolish. Thus, in the early nineteenth century, Hale underwent an intravenous injection of half an ounce of castor oil. The only benefit that accrued from this undertaking was a vivid description of the severe reaction, which Hale happily survived (Macht, 1916).

Among the many carefully planned experiments performed upon the investigator himself are those of such men as Head and Bichat (Jefferson, 1955) who mutilated themselves in an effort to elucidate the anatomy and physiology of sensory nerves, and of Forssmann, who laid the groundwork for important advances in the understanding of the circulatory phenomena by threading a long catheter into his own right ventricle (Forssmann, 1929). Such experiments involving only one subject have produced many important advances in medical science

Often in experimental studies small groups of trained observers have been utilized as subjects, usually including the investigator or investigators themselves. Notable in this category are the studies of body metabolism by Eugene DuBois (DuBois, 1948) and the research on pain by Sir Thomas Lewis and his group (Lewis, 1942), James Hardy, Harold Wolff, and Helen Goodell (Hardy et al., 1952).[5]

Volunteers

A great many experiments have been performed on healthy "volunteer" subjects. The use of volunteers for medical study involves not only the problem of appropriate selection, but it also raises important ethical questions. Some such studies, especially those involving preventive procedures, have had potential benefit for the subjects involved. Following the interest of Lady Wortley Montagu in smallpox inoculation, George I of England arranged for experimental smallpox inoculation of six so-called volunteer prisoners who had been condemned to death. There followed a second experiment on several poor children. Since all the subjects remained well, King George arranged for his own children to be inoculated (Bett, 1954). Less colorful, perhaps, but more extensive studies have been done with human volunteer subjects using gamma globulin and Salk vaccine against polio (Spencer, 1953; Hammon et al. 1952).

Many experiments performed on human volunteers have not involved any potential benefit, but rather a potential hazard to the subject. Thus, during World War II, a great many subjects exposed themselves to infectious hepatitis and serum hepatitis (Drake, 1952; Mirick et al., 1954; Henle, 1950; Stokes, 1954) as well as the common cold (Andres, 1953), cat scratch fever (Blattner & Heyes, 1956), scrub typhus (Spencer, 1953), murine typhus (Wolbach et al., 1922) and a variety of other infections. Precedence for these studies derived from work with measles as early as 1759, when Home inoculated twelve children with material from patients with measles and observed that seven of them developed the disease (Spencer, 1953). Later, Steiner (1875), Hektoen, and others (Hiro & Tasaka, 1938) reported similar experiences, but doubtless the best known experiments dealing with human volunteers in relation to infectious diseases were those of Walter Reed and his colleagues, who allowed themselves to be bitten by infected mosquitos (Kelly, 1906). Later, Gorgas and his collaborators made a similar experiment in the case of malaria (Gorgas, 1918) and in 1923 Dicks produced scarlet fever by inoculating human volunteers with streptococci (Grant, 1953). The prophylaxis for syphilis that commanded such enormous interest at the turn of the century was achieved by Metchnikoff, who was able to prevent the disease by the use of calomel ointment prior to the experimental infection of a human volunteer (Haggard, 1929).

Striking among the aspects of experiments performed on human volunteers is the great variability in the degree to which the submission is voluntary. Sometimes, as in the case of conscientious objectors during wartime (*Time Magazine*, 1945) a subject's motivations may be very complicated indeed. Medical and dental students have provided a consistent source of so called volunteers for research. Usually they are paid or are rewarded by symbols of approval. Prisoners participating in medical research are likely to achieve some sort of special consideration, often not great. Ninety years ago, R.P. Strong used prisoners condemned to death for a study of the plague (Strong, 1906). His prisoners received an extra piece of tobacco as compensation. Sometimes experiments have been done on prisoners without their knowledge; thus, a helminthologist once gave a condemned woman the larvae of intestinal worms shortly before her execution. This was done in order to determine whether or not the worms developed in the intestines after death. Later, convicts in the Ohio State Penitentiary were injected with living cancer cells (*Science News Letter*, 1957).

Much experimentation has been wholly involuntary on the part of the subject, as in the case of the victims of the Nazis. Claude Bernard has provided an account of the kings of Prussia having delivered to physicians men condemned to death in order to perform vivisections on them that might be useful to science, and added that according to Galen, Attalus III, c. 137 B.C., experimented with poisons and antidotes on criminals who were condemned to die (Bernard, 1926). The contributions of patient-subjects have often been immortalized in the medical literature. The blood groups, Kell, Duffy, and Kidd were named for the patients in whom they were discovered and it was a sick patient under study, not a season, that supplied the colorful name for the variant of hemophilia called Christmas disease (Witts, 1955).

Patients Participating in Clinical Research

There are several ways in which patients are used in experimental research. First, subjects with unusual defects or deformities may be studied. The most classical example is the work of William Beaumont on his fistulous subject, Alexis St. Martin (Beaumont, 1833) studies which demonstrated that numbers are not indispensable to progress in research. Patients with unique deformities or defects have contributed enormously to our understanding of physiology and physiopathology; so have those with surgically produced defects. The work of Foerster in mapping sensory pathways is notable in this regard (Jefferson, 1955). Here there has occasionally been a conflict of motivation on the part of the investigator, between providing relief for his patient and exploiting the opportunity to probe the unknown.

A second category in which patients are used for research includes those on whom a new therapy or maneuver is being tried in the hope of improving their condition. Again, some of these have been more hazardous than others. The feeding of liver by Minot and Murphy that resulted in an important advance in therapeutics was certainly tedious but not dangerous (Minot & Murphy, 1927). The use of estrogenic hormones in the prophylaxis of coronary artery disease (Stamler et al., 1956) was conceivably hazardous, but many procedures undertaken with the hope of bringing individual benefit to the patient have offered much more immediate hazards. These include lobotomy and related procedures, focal resections of the cortex in the treatment of epilepsy, hypophysectomy, and adrenalectomy for cancer, severe diabetes, or hypertension, and the great variety of surgical procedures on the heart. Other measures such as malaria in the treatment of general paresis, insulin coma, metrazol shock or electroshock treatment in psychoses must have seemed very hazardous indeed when they were first tried. So also must be the first blood transfusion performed by Denis in 1666 (Denis, 1667), or the first use of anesthesia in surgery or hypnotism as an anesthetic maneuver (Garrison, 1929), or the first use of diphtheria antitoxin, (Wernicke, 1913) or the dramatic treatment of nine-year-old Joseph Miester, who had been bitten by a rabid dog and to whom Pasteur gave his first prophylactic serum treatment (Rapport & Wright, 1952).

Another category of patients used in experimental research includes those who are hopelessly ill or moribund and who become subjects for seriously risky procedures that may or may not have any direct relevance to their condition. Work of this type has been criticized from the ethical standpoint by such men as Ivy (1948), Wright (1956) and Sendrail (1954).

General Considerations Governing
Human Participation as Subjects

Strict ethical standards for research on humans have been imposed during the past fifteen years by institutional review boards required in every medical research institution. There must be full disclosure of the procedures to be undertaken and the potential hazards that might be involved. There must also be informed consent by the patient and patient-subjects with firm assurance that they may withdraw from the experiment at any time that they may choose to do so.

Among subjects for clinical research are patients who happen to be conveniently accessible as subjects because of being in a hospital, but for whom the experiments have no direct relevance. Here problems of selection and adequate design have plagued the investigator. Matching as to age, sex, and even genetic and constitutional composition may not be enough. The very fact of their being a captive group makes them susceptible to certain symbolic stimuli arising out of personal interactions on the ward (Schottstaedt et al., 1954). Also, simply being bedfast, may seriously skew the data from hemodynamic studies and even metabolic data may be altered by inactivity. Other factors of selection can also limit the usefulness of certain humans as subjects. Failure to take cognizance of a skewed selection may vitiate inferences drawn from the studies. The validity of the human sample must be separately established for nearly every type of study. For example, if the circumstances of the experiment happened to be frightening enough to a particular group of people, one might adduce convincing evidence in a thousand subjects that an inert agent induced tachycardia, anorexia, or urinary frequency.

The difficulty of obtaining an adequate sample of human subjects that will allow for inferences concerning the effects of pharmacodynamic agents has been pointed out by Lasagna and associates, who observed that college students who required a financial inducement for "volunteering" to participate in a series of drug-testing experiments were emotionally more maladjusted than were a group of healthy subjects of comparable size who had requested no emolument (Lasagna, 1954).

Poor experimental control is well illustrated by a study of the results of the thoracolumbar sympathectomy for essential hypertension. The group used to control the experiment consisted of patients carefully matched to the operated group as to age, sex, duration, and severity of the disease, but who had refused operation when recommended (Smithwick, 1951). A high degree of selection is implied here in terms of the general attitude and adaptability of the patient and of the quality of the doctor-patient relationship. Often in a therapeutic experiment, critical factors of selection have not been apparent until long after the studies were completed.

Even when selection has been faultless, serious errors may result from failure to appreciate that the circumstances of the experiment and its significance to the patient may exert important effects. it has been abundantly shown that numerous bodily organs and organ systems are capable of responding in a major way to situations because of their meaning (Wolff et al., 1949).

Experimental Design

There are no universally applicable rules-of-thumb for proper design in clinical research. Each inquiry demands its own tailor-made rules to assiduously avoid the trap so aptly described by MacCaulay where "the inquiry may amuse us, but the description leaves us no wiser" (Witts, 1955). The difficulty is in knowing what needs to be controlled. The quality of the investigation and of its research design are of the first importance, but it is well to remember that, brilliant as the ideas may be and assiduous the workers, the indispensable element in clinical research is the contribution of the patients who submit to studies and who thereby become our partners in research.

Ethics and Civility in Research

Medical research is always a shared undertaking. No matter how brilliant is the investigator's concept, how skillful his inquiry or how elegant his evidence, he is not working alone. Not only are his students and his helpers indispensable, but so are the insights and achievements of his predecessors.

Acknowledgement of the work of those investigators who have gone before is mandatory. We all build on a structure that has been erected by our forebears in science. Many of the bibliographies in reports of current research have not only ignored signal contributions of previous workers, but reviews have taken on the flavor of original contributions with inadequate acknowledgement of original data from competing contemporary scientists.

Bibliographic citations are intended to inform a journal's readers of the details of methods used or to provide them additional information on topics covered in the articles. The most civilized purpose of citations, however, is the acknowledgement of priority for an original idea or discovery. Unfortunately, this proper use of citations seems to have become a casualty of World War II as postwar medical journals proliferated and editors vied with one another for prestige. One of the procrustean demands was that the citations in submitted articles be up to date. Even the reviewers often commented unfavorably if most of an author's citations were not of very recent vintage. As a consequence, authors have frequently committed the indignity of citing recent reviews of a topic rather than original reports.

Ironically, with citations to original work appearing less and less frequently in bibliographies, they have begun to serve as a gauge of the worth of young scientists. Thanks to the ease with which citations can be collected and listed by computer, they are continuously harvested and periodically published as the authoritative *Citation Index.* Unfortunately there has been a loosening of moral fiber among those engaged in medical research. There have been several instances of falsification of data since shortly after the Vietnam war. This new threat to science has become so troublesome that the National Institutes of Health have been required to establish a bureau to deal with fraud in research.

Notes

1. The Gilles de la Tourette syndrome is characterized by uncoordinated movements of the extremities and of the structures responsible for speech. It was originally recognized in 1825, was described again in 1880 but the first complete account was delineated by the French neurologist Gilles de la Tourette in 1885. Onset is in childhood, usually before the age of ten.
2. According to Franklin H. Portugal and Jack S. Cohen, Griffith was "an immensely dedicated scientist—a virtual recluse known to only a few associates. His dedication cost him his life. During the blitz in London in 1941, Griffith was killed while working in his laboratory." Whether or not he would have ultimately determined that his transforming factor was DNA one can only speculate.
3. Altschule, a highly individualistic teacher at Harvard, was viewed by the students as an icon among the faculty. He taught that the important aim of a clinical evaluation was "to understand the patient's message," however it was conveyed.
4. William Beaumont, an American army surgeon stationed at Mackinac Island, Michigan, was called to treat a young man, Alexis St. Martin, who had sustained an accidental bullet wound to his abdomen that left a channel from his stomach lining through to an opening in his abdominal wall. After years of study of St. Martin's stomach, Beaumont in 1833 published the book, *Observations on the Gastric Juice and the Physiology of Digestion*, soon to become an enduring classic of medical research.
5. In these and subsequent studies, heart rate variability was calculated from measurement of the mean rate and standard deviation or by spectral analysis. In 1990 James Skinner and collaborators, using the point correlation dimension of chaos theory, developed a more precise and definitive method of predicting sudden arrhythmic death by measurements of heart rate variability (Skinner et al., 1990).
6. The average human subject is not usually capable of estimating the intensity of a sensation with much consistency while these investigators were able to sharpen the perceptions of their subjects by training so that they could reliably recall the intensity of stimuli from test to test.

5

Financing Medical Research

The Private Foundations

Prior to 1950 medical research was supported almost entirely from private or commercial philanthropy. Among private foundations were The Medical Board of the Rockefeller Foundation directed by Dr. Alan Gregg, a man of extraordinary intellectual cultivation, insight and judgment. With full authority to approve grants, he traveled to research laboratories throughout the United States, the British Isles and Commonwealth, and Europe, met personally with the investigators and witnessed their work. He promised support to those who passed muster and, as he left their laboratories, he would say, "Don't send me any reports. Send me the reprints." Several other major foundations that supported research in American universities at that time also operated in a personal and nonbureaucratic fashion. Among them were the R.H. Macy Foundation, the Commonwealth Fund, the John A. Hartford Foundation, Inc., Albert and Mary Lasker Foundation, Inc., the Helen Hay Whitney Foundation, Inc., and the Pew Memorial Trust.

The Birth of the NIH

The National Institutes of Health grew from a small hygiene laboratory of the U.S. Public Health Service established in New York in 1888. Three years later it was moved to Washington as a research resource for training young Public Health officers under the directorship of Dr. Milton Rosenau. Among his students were many individuals who later assumed leadership posts in medical schools and research institutes across the country. The NIH as we know it was established in 1948 on land presented to the government by Mr. and Mrs. Luke I. Wilson in Bethesda,

Maryland. The new National Institutes of Health included the already existing National Cancer Institute, established by Congress in 1937, and the newly created National Heart Institute and the National Institute for Dental Research. By then an extramural granting program had become well established.

Financial support for medical researchers was also available from some pharmaceutical companies mainly for therapeutic studies. Costs for research were not large at that time. Many investigators fashioned their own instruments. Neither computers nor high-tech electronics, ultrasound, radioactive markers nor nuclear magnetic resonance imaging techniques had become available.

Following World War II, there was a sharp increase in applicants for medical school thanks to the financial support offered by the G.I. Bill of Rights. There also occurred an explosive increase in the availability of antibiotics, especially penicillin, and new tools for medical research, diagnosis, and treatment. Medical schools across the country expanded and modernized, welcoming to their faculties young medical scientists and teachers trained mainly in the eastern universities. This expansion of academic medicine made evident the need for new sources of financial support for medical research.

Accordingly, under the leadership of Dr. Joseph Hinsey, a distinguished neurophysiologist and professor of anatomy at Cornell Medical College in New York City, representatives from several institutions met with the leaders of large industrial firms. The heads of many of these industries were persuaded to assign 5 percent of their net profits to support medical research, with funds to be managed by a suitable representative foundation.

This bold plan was moving close to realization when Mrs. Mary Lasker, wife of a wealthy advertising executive in Chicago began to turn the tide toward federal government support. With the help of Senator Lister Hill and representative John E. Fogarty of Delaware, she and a group of interested colleagues convinced President Truman and the Congress to make the National Institutes of Health the prime support for medical research in American and to convert the National Institute of Health into several institutes responsible for providing support for research in each of the major disease areas of the nation. There are now seventeen such institutes plus supporting agencies. The first director of the National Institutes of Health, Dr. Rolla E. Dyer, an expert in tropical medicine and epidemiology, was succeeded in 1950 by a famous nutritionist,

Dr. William H. Sebrell, Jr. who, in 1955 was succeeded by Dr. James A. Shannon who served until 1968. The NIH established the preeminence of the United States in the support of biomedical research. Most worthy research proposals were funded at that time and scientific productivity sprang up in universities and institutes all over the country.

During the first few succeeding years, when the appropriations from Congress amounted to less than 1 billion dollars, the business of financing research was left pretty well to the director, Dr. James Shannon. He worked closely with Senator Lister Hill, Representative Fogarty, Mary Lasker, Florence Maloney, and several other lay supporters who helped persuade congress to provide increasing support to the NIH.

These were the halcyon days of medical research in the United States. The NIH programs were administered not by bureaucrats but by dedicated servants of the mission. The administrative staff was small. The public health officers charged with management were frequently heard to declare, "This is the scientists' program, our task is to expedite their efforts." Such words were uttered by the principle officers of the NIH such as Cassius Van Slyke, Franklin Yeager, Ralph Knutti, James Shannon, and others. The extraordinary competence of these people and the effective way in which they spent the public's money, moved Dr. Lewis Thomas to declare the NIH: "the most brilliant social invention of the twentieth century."

There were, of course, turf battles among the various component institutes. Congress enhanced the programs of heart, cancer, and mental health. Appropriations continued to increase thanks to the efforts of Mary Lasker and her colleagues which were implemented by persuasive lobbying from the universities. Support was so strong that an office of international research was created to support rapidly emerging new research from Europe, Israel, and a few countries elsewhere.[1] Shortly after the budget of the NIH had reached 1 billion dollars senators and members of Congress began to demand special NIH support for certain specific diseases affecting their constituents.

A very unfortunate perturbation of the system occurred during the spring of 1964. Representative Lawrence H. Fountain of North Carolina announced in Congress that a certain institution that had been funded for research had used a small amount of the money to entertain visiting lecturers at dinner. This seemingly minor episode, widely reported in the press, triggered a typically costly bureaucratic response.[2] Rules and guidelines, along with their inevitable paper work were drawn up for grantee institutions who, at first, were required to make their own detailed financial reports, but soon NIH employees were detailed to the institutions to work in their offices to monitor financial records.

Congress became more and more participatory in regulating the NIH and, under pressure from their constituents, began calling for more institutes and renaming some of the existing ones. As appropriations grew, rules and regulations proliferated and there was an explosive increase in the number of staff positions and a demand for space in which to locate them. In addition to the buildings on the NIH campus, therefore, NIH acquired or rented space in some dozens of additional buildings throughout Bethesda, Chevy Chase, and Washington. James Shannon fell ill and was succeeded by Dr. Robert Marston who in turn was succeeded by Dr. Robert Stone and four additional successors up to the present time.

By 1987 the NIH had become a large, impersonal, costly government bureau with a congressional appropriation of 6.2 billion dollars of which only 50 percent was devoted to the support of investigator-initiated research. Therefore, instead of being able to support the "scientists' program" in line with the original NIH staff's declared mission, the currently available funds can support only 10 to 15 percent of the approved research applications from individual scientists.

Unfortunately, in the face of this serious shortage of support for creative medical research in the U.S. there has been no widespread effort on the part of private foundations to compensate for the deficiency. Instead, the programs of most of the large foundations are now focused on social causes, highly worthy and in need of support, but in the meantime other parts of the world, including several European countries and Japan which offer strong support for their scientists, are rapidly moving into the forefront of innovative medical research. Especially deprived of support has been clinical investigation, the research concerned with human health and disease in which the human beings themselves are the subjects of investigation (Ahrens, 1992). In his book, *The Crisis in Clinical Research* Ahrens recounts the metamorphosis of the NIH from servant of medical science to arbiter of what kind of research should be recognized and awarded support. Such judgments, made at the various administrative levels, have poured disproportionately large sums into research on a single disease, AIDS, implicating a virus without its contribution to the cause having been firmly established.[3] Ever larger sums have been poured into the effort to identify all of the genes among human chromosomes despite the fact that the number of clearly genetically determined diseases is small, less than 2 percent. Furthermore, in those diseases in which the relevant gene has been isolated and identified, that knowledge has not as yet offered any new useful therapy. For example, the gene responsible for sickle cell anemia and that responsible for Huntington's chorea were identified more than twenty years ago without a useful clue to therapy having as yet emerged.

Medical research, like other human activities, is partly governed by fashion, by what others are endorsing and doing. Other inappropriate determining factors are uninformed emotionally based requirements imposed by the Congress, political influence from industrial interests, and preferences determined by the NIH institutes themselves.

It is only fair to say that the climate in which medical research is presently supported and performed is far less salubrious than it was fifty years ago. A small percentage of productive investigators can obtain support and only a minority (less than 30 percent) of today's NIH funded investigators have had a medical education. The criteria used by "peer" reviewers in study sections are increasingly focused on the form and minute detail of a proposal and its adherence to accepted dogma rather than its bold insight, originality and the "track record" of the applicant.

The task of the responsible authorities is clearly to reexamine and recast the entire process of supplying financial support for medical research. The current level of congressional appropriation would probably suffice if headquarters and operational expenditures were pared down, the administrative staff sharply reduced and the administrative prerogatives reduced to expediting instead of prescribing the projects of the scientists.

Notes

1. Fellowships for foreign students to work at U.S. institutions comprised a major part of the program. It also supported a few American students for work in European laboratories. Project support for principal investigators in foreign laboratories was also provided. Visits to the laboratories and to the research fellows in training were made periodically by NIH consultants stationed in London, Paris and elsewhere. The program was almost abandoned during the latter years of the 1960s because of increasing financial demands from U.S. institutions.
2. Oversight of accounting at the grantee institutions was intensified and administrative regulation was increased in other ways, including monitoring the race and gender distribution of human subjects for research, facilities for experimental animals, etc. The NIH maintains separate bureaus for protection from research

risks, for research on women's health, for the investigation of research integrity, for grant inquiries, for science policy and legislation, and so on. This vast administrative expansion and the welter of publications and correspondence that emerge from the various bureaucratic units has occasioned an impressive increase in the number of NIH employees and in the cost of the space they occupy and the resources they use. By 1989 the Congressional appropriation to NIH had reached eight billion dollars, twenty-five percent of which was spent on administrative functions.

3. The NIH support for AIDS research amounted to $1,300,000,000.00 in 1994. Since the appearance of AIDS on the medical scene in 1981 federal support for research into cause, treatment, and prevention has failed to yield a clear understanding of cause, a useful and safe treatment, or an effective means of prevention beyond the obvious simple prudent avoidance of promiscuous sexual intercourse and of contaminated needles. The former hazard of contaminated blood from blood banks is now extremely low.

By 1989 the annual Congressional appropriation to NIH had reached eight billion dollars, twenty-five percent of which was spent on administrative functions.

4. The NIH support for AIDS research amounted to $1,300,000,000.00 in 1994. Since the appearance of AIDS on the medical scene in 1981 federal support for research into cause, treatment, and prevention has failed to yield a clear understanding of cause, a useful and safe treatment, or an effective means of prevention beyond the obvious simple prudent avoidance of promiscuous sexual intercourse and of contaminated needles. The former hazard of contaminated blood from blood banks is now extremely low.

6

Determinants of Health and Disease

Searching for a Cause

The traditional line of inquiry in the study of disease has been to seek ultimate causes. In the sixteenth century, Jean Fernel wrote, "Misbalance of the Constitution is the illness, yet the cause is the practical point. There are causes we do not know" (Sherrington, 1946). The concept of "cause" has undergone radical change from era to era in medicine until today the search for a single cause has been all but abandoned. In its place we have the currently popular concept of multicausality of diseases, something resembling Fernel's "misbalance." It recognizes that the number of ways things can go wrong is less than the number of things that can perturb the bodily economy. It also takes into account the myriad regulatory mechanisms of the body, disruptions of which are manifested as diseases (Wolf, 1963).

While microbes and toxins are numbered among the agents of disease, in most instances it is the body's response that constitutes the manifestations of disease, as vividly demonstrated by Rowe, who irradiated mice to impair their lymphocyte response to injection of the virus of lymphocytic chloriomenengitis. Without preliminary radiation, all animals sickened and nearly all died. The irradiated animals, on the other hand, were actually protected against any evidence of illness but, nevertheless, they continued to harbor the virus (Rowe, 1956). There are many other examples showing that infectious diseases represent not so much the depredations of the invader as they do the adaptations of the host: the tubercle in tuberculosis, for example, and the precipitated antigen-antibody complex in the glomerular tuft in Bright's disease are the product of the defensive behavior of the body.

Since the variety of possible adaptations is limited, the same types of molecular and cellular reactions show up in various parts of the body as pathogenic mechanisms or conditions that we designate as separate diseases. Today more attention is paid to the disturbed regulatory processes than to the naming of diseases. Such regulatory disturbances responsible for the manifestations of various diseases can be triggered or augmented, or perhaps inhibited by a variety of external forces, by individual behaviors, and even by the way a person interprets or deals with his human relationships and life experiences.

With respect to cause, man, over the course of recorded history, has vacillated between placing the blame on outside hostile forces and on himself. One hundred years ago the work of Pasteur made it appear that the question was settled decisively in favor of the outside forces, and yet even as Pasteur was inducted into the French Academy, his opponent, Pidoux, objected that, "disease is the common result of a variety of diverse external and internal causes [that] bring about the destruction of an organ by a number of roads which the hygienist and the physician must endeavor to close" (Pidoux, 1959).

Concerning cause we seemed to be on firm ground when Rudolf Virchow, examining stained slices of tissue through his microscope, was becoming the father of cellular pathology. Virchow's formulations suggested that each causative agent in disease produces a specific and identifiable tissue change. For a good many years thereafter physicians operated on the assumption that the proper cause of each disease could be identified by a microscope of sufficiently high power and an adequate variety of staining techniques. Today, however, we realize that there are only a limited number of tissue responses in the face of myriad noxious agents causing disease.

In such diseases as essential hypertension, peptic ulcer, and ulcerative colitis where no specific etiologic agent has been identified, preoccupation with cause gives way to a consideration of mechanisms and of factors capable of setting them in motion. From such inquiry has emerged the realization that most diseases classified as involving one organ or organ system actually produce a widespread integrated set of bodily changes that may include several organs and organ systems. In pneumonia, for example, there is consolidation of the lung that consists of the alveolar spaces being filled with partially coagulated fluid and a few white and red blood cells. The capillaries in the alveolar septa are dilated, presumably a vasomotor effect. In addition, white cells are manufactured at a greatly increased rate in the relatively distant bone marrow. The lymph nodes or other parts of the reticuloendothelial system produce antibodies, and, of course, the brain itself has its temperature regulating equipment readjusted to produce fever. The whole process of bringing these widely scattered mechanisms into play is delicately timed and executed in an orderly way. Pneumonia, more than being just a pulmonary disease, is an integrated response of the body as a whole.

At this moment we have strong experimental evidence indicating that many of the component changes in disease processes, including fever, leucocytosis, headache, nausea, and alterations in vasomotor, glandular, smooth muscle, and mucous membrane function may be set in motion by impulses arising in the cerebral cortex. Such messages from the forebrain appear to be initiated in response to afferent signals from the body itself or from the environment via the special sensory structures. The influence of the forebrain on the manifestations of disease have been vividly demonstrated in experimental studies of disorders manifested by nasal congestion, skin rashes, stomach, duodenal, and bladder contraction, esophageal obstruction, colon behavior, heartbeat, and kidney impairment (Wolff, 1952; Wolf & Goodell, 1975). Evidence of disease may be elicited by infectious agents, by ocean travel, offensive odors, or by irrigating one external auditory canal with cold water, or may occur in response to neural activity in the forebrain elicited by language symbols and other situational stimuli without the subject necessarily being consciously aware of being emotionally stressed. A simple illustration of such unconscious receptor activity occurs when one is using a monocular microscope with both eyes held open. The experienced microscopist quickly learns to blot out from consciousness the image that appears on the retina of the eye which is not looking in the ocular, even though the electrical impulses set up in the optic nerve are doubtless carried through the usual pathways to the receptive areas of the occipital cortex.

Infectious Diseases

In 1884, just a few years after the revolutionary findings of Pasteur and Koch, the American Clinical and Climatological Association came into being because the founders were not convinced that microbes explained everything about such diseases as tuberculosis, the leading scourge of those days. Koch's identification of the tubercle bacillus was well known to them, but they could not believe that the microbes alone determined either the pathogenesis of or recovery from the disease. On the other hand, differences in geographical distribution of the prevalence and severity of tuberculosis directed the attention of climatologists to the physical ambience, air, temperature, and moisture, so they devoted much of their meetings to a consideration of the curative powers of spas and resorts.

Some years later, René Dubos, who spent much of his scientific life in pursuit of the tubercle bacillus, called attention to the fact that, while the presence of the tubercle bacillus is essential to the occurrence of tuberculous infection, it has little to do with determining the severity of the infection, or even whether or not infection will occur (Dubos, 1940). From his thorough studies of the relation between social order and disease he concluded that more significant than crowding, cold, malnutrition, and poor hygiene to the spread of tuberculosis was social upheaval. He did not dismiss such environmental forces as exposure to cold and rain, lack of food, excessive effort, crowding, and contact with a densely infected migratory population, but he placed more emphasis on the difficult social adjustments consequent upon migrations from rural to urban life and from one country to another during the nineteenth- and early twentieth-century industrialization. Mortality from tuberculosis reached its peak within ten to twenty years after industrialization began and thereafter fell off rapidly suggesting an intangible factor beyond the tangible hazards of industrialization (McDougal, 1949; Krause, 1928; Dubos, 1940). Further, Dubos reminded us that we create new diseases for ourselves as rapidly as we subdue some of the old ones (Dubos, 1959). The new diseases seemed to stem from the way we manipulate our environment, social as well as physical, and the way we react to the altered environment.[1]

Such a view was embodied in the ancient Chinese philosophy of Taoism, developed during the century before the birth of Christ. Disease was the result of man's being out of balance with his environment. Cure depended upon adjusting the relationship between Yin, the negative cosmic force, and Yang, the positive. Phenomena generally recognized as indications of disease include quantitative alterations in body temperature, arterial pressure, the formed elements of the blood, vasomotor activity and hemodynamic mechanisms, the secretory activity of glands, and certain biosynthetic functions as, for example, those that characterize the sequence of blood coagulation. Other manifestations of disease include vomiting, malaise, headache, and other pain; muscular weakness, alterations in mood and behavior, and loss of consciousness; alterations in the amount and composition of blood plasma, and excretory products; shifts in the concentration of various ions in cells and body compartments; immunological phenomena involving alterations in capillary permeability; excessive cell reproduction; and tissue changes such as hyperemia, edema, and necrosis. A great variety of diseases that share these features have been shown to be subject to influence or control by the central nervous system acting through neural, immunological, or endocrine pathways (Bykov, 1957; Speransky, 1953; Rushmer & Smith, 1959; Hoff and Green, 1936). Even potentially fatal cardiac arrhythmias that occur in association with myocardial infarction are actuated by forebrain circuits (Skinner, 1993).

Human Nature as a Biological Mechanism

In one species of spider the female, after laying her eggs, stands by and watches until the eggs hatch. Often enough, by the time they have hatched, she has been without food for so long that she dies in the effort to get the next meal. It is clear from this and other evidence that the responsibility of a parent for her young is "built into the organism," or instinctive if you wish. Such behavior has the same biological validity throughout the animal kingdom and in man. It is important, however, that the spider's behavioral control is "hard wired," while the human's behavior is contingent upon choice, nonlinear. The human infant may or may not be nourished and cared for. Nevertheless, irrespective of the degree of motivation, the mother-love behavior is so useful and in the best interest of the race of spiders and the race of man that during the course of evolution it has become a part of the nature of the spider and of man. Humans are less consistent in their behavior than spiders. Their decision to care for the young or not to do so is governed by equipment not available to a spider, a personal value system involving moral convictions, preferences, and personal affinities. As with other biological mechanisms, a choice of behavior eventually tends to become stereotyped. We are likely to reenact our characteristic patterns of behavior over and over until they become so characteristic that friends may recognize us by them. For example, when threatened or put in a tight corner, the cautious man becomes more cautious; the gambler takes a gamble; the fighter fights; and the fleer flees. We may argue the degree to which these characteristic patterns of behavior are innate or inborn, but we could not argue whether or not they are biological. It would appear, then, that making decisions is certainly as biological as making tears or generating rapid heart beats. When a situation arouses delight, or displeasure, the consequent response depends on how the event is perceived and evaluated in the brain. Such cortical neuronal decision making may elicit changes in endocrine, immunological, and enzyme systems that when intense or prolonged, may become manifest as disease.

The Integrated Multisystem Participation in Disease Processes

Traditionally, physicians have been inclined to consider diseases to be more localized than they really are, often on the spurious assumption that they involve only a single organ or organ system. Thus, pneumonia is thought of as a disease of the lungs although many of its manifestations—including fever, leucocytosis, increased antibody titers, tachycardia, and so on—are brought about by changes in organs distant from the lungs, such as the brain, the bone marrow, the lymph nodes, and the heart. In congestive heart failure, for example, delicately balanced chemical, circulatory, and renal adjustments are well known as well as several alterations in endocrine secretions, including the antidiuretic hormone, aldosterone, thyroid hormone, and corticosteroids. Again, all of these regulatory mechanisms have been shown to be connected with and responsive to the central nervous system.

Recognizing the importance of adaptation to health, J.B.S. Haldane (Haldane, 1935) declared: "Progress in medicine depends on understanding how the human organism adapts to changes in his environment." I would further suggest that the adaptations of the human organism, when exaggerated, insufficient, or inappropriate in some way actually *constitute* the manifestations of disease.

For example, a healthy person living at a high altitude, as in the Andes, maintains a substantially elevated red blood cell count, thereby compensating for the diminished atmospheric pressure of oxygen. The additional red cells are needed to deliver adequate oxygen to the tissues. When such a rise in a red cell count occurs at sea level, however, the increase is inappropriate and a disease, polycythemia, is present. The bodily mechanisms required to increase the number of circulating red blood cells are, nevertheless, identical in both situations, in health and in disease. As another example, a heart rate of 120 in a runner immediately after a 100-yard dash would be considered a sign of health, but in a sedentary patient the same heart rate would be a clear evidence of illness.

Environment and Metabolism

Some years ago, Dr. William Schottstaedt and I studied the impact of a social environment on the metabolism of human subjects who were resident on a research ward. The experimental design included analysis of several metabolites from day to day in the urine and feces of the patients. While their diet and exercise were kept uniform (Schottstaedt et al., 1958, 1959, 1963). Throughout the period of study the social interactions of the long-term inhabitants of the ward were recorded by the doctors, nurses, and a participant observer whose presence was not known to the patients who varied in number from fifteen to twenty during the study period. Those responsible for recording behavior and emotional responses were kept ignorant of the laboratory findings.

We found that the ward had the special characteristics of a well-defined community with its own pressures, values, prestige points, and taboos. In short, it had established its own social equilibrium. Even transient disruptions of the equilibrium were associated with substantial measurable metabolic changes.

Major metabolic changes in terms of urinary excretion of water, sodium, potassium, calcium, nitrogen, and creatinine occurred repeatedly in situations of stress among the patients (table 6.3). Deviations in excretion of metabolites of greater than two standard deviations occurred on sixty of a total of 213 patient-days for which data were available. The metabolic deviations correlated with the prevailing atmosphere of the ward: many more occurred when the ward community as a whole was disrupted.

Eighty-six percent of stressful events were accompanied by significant alterations in the balance data when the atmosphere of the ward was disturbed, while during relatively calm periods for the group as a whole only 48 percent of episodes rated as stressful were accompanied by significant changes. "False positives," or metabolic deviations of signifi-

Table 6.1
Stresses Occurring on a Metabolic Ward

	Quiet	Disturbed	Total
Stressful days on which metabolic data were available	25	42	67
Non-stressful days on which metabolic data were available	78	68	146
Total patient-days on which metabolic data were available	103	110	213
Stressful days with significant metabolic deviations	12	36	48
Non-stressful days with significant metabolic deviations	7	5	12
% of stressful days with significant metabolic deviations	48	86	72
% of non-stressful days with significant metabolic deviations	9	7	8

cant degree, occurred on only twelve of 146 patient-days (8 percent) that had not been independently judged as stressful.

Interpersonal difficulties among those with strong ties were much the most common sources of stress to be associated with metabolic deviations, accounting for twenty-eight of the forty-six stressful situations associated with such deviations. Interpersonal stresses arising between individuals without strong ties were less often associated with significant changes in the metabolic data.

Configuration vs. Quantitation of Data

When the nurses on the ward were asked to submit to a psychological testing procedure and to evaluate the performance of one another in relating to individual patients, they proved to be reluctant and personally threatened by the request. The atmosphere of the ward for the next several days was tense and subdued. Throughout this period of uneasiness, all of the patients under study on the ward displayed a uniform metabolic response consisting of a negative balance of all measured metabolites, even though the patients were unaware of the circumstances responsible for the nurses' anxiety. This experience illustrates that a bodily response to stress depends not so much on the *quantity* of the noxious stimulus but rather on the quality or *configuration* of the prevailing circumstances. Thus, looking only for quantifiable data may cause one to miss the most pertinent evidence.

A vivid example of the importance of configuration in biology is evident in the contrast of smell and taste between the enantiomers (isomers) spearmint and caraway (Russell, 1971). Shapes and electrical changes are now explaining the action of many molecules in a way that a knowledge of their quantitative composition could never do. In medicine we are just beginning to learn to relegate our preoccupation with quantitation to its proper place and also to ask configurational questions in more than one dimension. The configuration or pattern of an individual's adaptive response to a meaningful circumstance depends first of all on perception, beyond that on the interpretative process in the brain, and finally on the response of the neural control mechanisms that govern physiological and general behavior.

Neural Adaptations

We now have ample evidence that the immunologic, metabolic, and vascular adjustments that adapt an individual to his environment are regulated by an extensive hierarchy of chemical and electrical mechanisms that encompass the whole range from local responses to supratentorial commands. Too many or too few of such adaptive responses or their inappropriate use constitutes, as has already been mentioned, the very manifestations of disease. Since, when Ling and Gerard (1949) recorded action potentials from inside a single muscle fiber and later, when J.C. Eccles recorded from single neurons in the central nervous system, technologic development in the study of the circuitry of the brain and the relationship of brain mechanisms to behavior has been so rapid as to be dizzying. A major part of the advance has consisted of the identification, localization, and manipulation of neurotransmitters and the clear demonstration of the importance of inhibitory systems in the overall process of human behavior regulation.

As more and more has been learned about facilitatory and inhibitory regulation of synaptic transmission at every level of the nervous system, the concept of reflex control of visceral function has given way to a concept of neural interaction in which virtually all parts of the nervous and endocrine systems are interconnected and interactive, so that local perturbations may have widespread effects. Studies have clearly revealed that the somatic and visceral pathways are not two systems after all, but a single system in a state of continuous dynamic interaction as behaviors are initiated, maintained, and modified.

Two Powerful and Long-Ignored Interactive Hormones

For more than twenty-five years, melatonin, the hormone of the pineal gland and dehydroepiandrosterone secreted by the adrenal cortex have been known about, and the structural formula for each of them had been identified. According to prevailing wisdom neither of them was considered to contribute in an important way to the bodily economy. While melatonin was acknowledged to play a role in controlling the timing of the twenty-four-hour sleep and wakefulness cycle, its main function was thought to have something to do with skin pigmentation. It does so in frogs, not in humans.

Dehydroepiandrosterone (DHEA and its sulfated twin, DHEAS) were thought to contribute weak androgenic effects to ovarian secretions. Over the last three to four years there has occurred an explosion of interest in these two hormones which share many important functions.

The blood concentration of DHEA peaks at very high levels in man (1200 ug/DL at about age twenty-one and decreases up to a hundredfold during aging. This marked decline in DHEA levels with aging has led many investigators to suggest that the drop in DHEA levels is the cause of a number of undesirable effects of aging, including:

1. Gradual loss of sensitivity to the action of insulin, glucose intolerance, and vascular disease (Haffner et al., 1995).
2. Loss of ability to make helpful antibodies to flu and other vaccines (Daynes et al., 1993).
3. Increased autoantibodies causing autoimmune diseases (Daynes et al., 1993).
4. Muscle wasting and increased osteoporosis (Ershler, 1994).

Most of these deficiencies have been shown to be reversed by oral administration of DHEA.

A preliminary study of elderly individuals performed at Totts Gap has shown an improvement in diabetic manifestations and in strength and vitality. There has also been a notable reduction of pain in rheumatoid arthritis. No adverse effects of DHEA or melatonin supplementation were encountered. In one report of a six month crossover study, the blind administration of fifty mg of DHEA vs. placebo to thirteen male and seventeen female subjects from forty to seventy years of age found that there was a significant increase in serum insulin-like growth factor and a decrease in insulin-like growth factor binding protein, strongly suggesting a shift from a catabolic (breakdown) to an anabolic (build up) state. In addition, from the use of fifty mg of DHEA per day for three months, 84 percent of females and 67 percent of males treated reported an improvement in physical and psychological well being. No untoward effects were experienced or displayed. Particularly significant was the absence of elevation of female hormones, estrone or estradiol in females given DHEA supplements (Morales et al., 1994). In another study there was evidence that DHEA exerts a hypolipidemic effect and an inhibitory effect on platelet agreation and reduces hyperinsulinema (Nestler et al., 1992).

The other neglected hormone, melatonin, has also been noted to decrease in aged animals, and, in addition, to be a potent free radical scavenger, particularly against the hydroxyl free radical (OH) (Poeggler et al., 1993). Free radicals are thought to exert significant toxicity during aging and supplementation with melatonin at doses of three to ten mg per day may exert a protective effect against free radical damage (Reiter, 1994). In support of this thesis, it has been reported that either supplementation with melatonin or transplantation of pineal glands in rats results in prolongation of life by up to one-third. In particular, the transplantation of pineal glands has led to an increase in the number of thymic lymphocytes, which normally decrease in aged animals (Pierpaoli & Regelson, 1994).

Mode of Action

It is clear that the mode of action of DHEA is not known beyond the fact that it does not bind to the usual steroid receptor (Morales, 1994). Furthermore, DHEA and its sulfate are present in blood of young adults in concentrations a thousandfold greater than normal glucocorticoids or sex steroids. It follows that DHEA is likely to be a substrate for further unknown reactions producing derivatives of much greater potency and much greater specificity than are shown by DHEA itself. Dr. Henry A.

Lardy of the Enzyme Institute of the University of Wisconsin has synthesized over twenty-five metabolites of DHEA. Some of these metabolites, such as the 7 alpha hydroxy form of DHEA have a remarkable ability to stimulate T-lymphocyte growth, particularly in diseases where the immune system is severely compromised. The effects of these compounds deserve serious investigation.

DHEA has the ability to lessen insulin requirement and decrease blood glucose in diabetic patients although the mode of action of DHEA in blocking the exuberant hepatic formation of glucose is not known but once the site of the inhibition of gluconeogenesis is known, the treatment of the catabolic state associated with severe sepsis and mortality associated with the treatment of injury should be greatly improved.

DHEA and Melatonin in Brain

DHEA is clearly a major "neurosteroid" (Akwa, 1991) and melatonin also acts on specific brain receptors. Both agents exert a more generalized effect as free radical scavengers.

The often encountered ability of DHEA to improve a patient's sense of "well being" has yet to be explained. There is also fragmentary evidence of the ability of DHEA to retard the onset of the memory defects of Alzheimer's disease.

Modulation and Illness

As more and more is learned about the neuroregulation of bodily functions, the balance of excitatory and inhibitory influences, one is reminded of the yin and yang of the ancient Chinese.

A defective balance between excitatory and inhibitory mechanisms may be responsible for a multitude of disorders including pathologic aggressiveness, alcoholism, epilepsy, and visceral disturbances such as the almost continuous gastric secretion of hydrochloric acid and proteolytic enzymes characteristic of duodenal ulcer, the sustained contraction of initially normal arterioles in hypertension, or the exaggerated ratio of destruction vs. production of red blood cells in hemolytic anemia as well as aberrations in other bodily systems including the cardiac arrhythmias that lead to sudden death. Personal conflicts and powerful social forces are important sources of such disturbances.

An important modulator of aberrations in adaptive behavior of bodily organs is morale, a group phenomenon reflecting common purpose and implying mutual support and assigning to all members of the group a respected place in the scheme of things. Perhaps in future research, attention should be given to social forces that sustain, encourage, and provide emotional nourishment, thereby balancing or counteracting the effects of life stresses.

We are indebted to Hans Selye for the demonstration that the same bodily disturbance, functional and anatomical, and the same lesions can be produced by a variety of agents. He demonstrated that the same kind of tissue reaction may recur in response to a diversity of agents, including stimuli that emanate from the interpretative areas of the brain. For years, in keeping with the teachings of Rudolph Virchow, it was believed that there was a microscopically identifiable lesion associated with each disease, the tubercle in tuberculosis, the Aschoff bodies for rheumatic fever, and so on. Selye's contribution was to show that identical tissue changes may be produced by a variety of stimuli, "stressors" of all sorts, physical, chemical, and symbolic from adverse life experience, all sharing the same underlying biological mechanisms.

Early workers in the field of emotion and disease such as Walter Cannon, had a unitary concept that held that emotionally stressful events are mediated by the sympathetic nerves affecting the body in a characteristic way: raising the blood sugar, increasing the output of epinephrine, quickening the pulse or stopping the activity of the digestive tract.

This now appears to be just part of the story. Emotionally charged situations may, for example, not only reduce, but also may increase the activity of the digestive tract. So may various other organs and their secretions become over- or underactive, in response to meaningful events. The face may either blush or turn pale, the bladder may become paralyzed or be overactive, and so on. (Wolf, 1968).

Awareness or lack of awareness of a situational conflict or an emotion is not essential to the occurrence of the response. In fact, the most powerful adverse experiences may be suppressed beyond recall. We have documented responses to both conscious and unconscious conflict situations involving virtually every organ of the body: eyes, skin, stomach, colon, heart, bladder, kidneys, etc. (Wolf, 1961). All of these structures are, of course, connected with and capable of reacting to regulatory influences from the interpretative areas of the brain. Thus, stressful stimuli do not need to reach awareness in order to have an effect. It is therefore a misnomer to state that emotion causes a bodily reaction since the reaction may occur without any awareness of emotion. It results from the processing of the experience by the brain by means of complex integrated interactions in neuronal circuits as they access stored information from previous life experience.

Man and His Brain

Presumably the high development of the mammalian nervous system has been responsible for the continued presence of our class in the world. The dinosaurs had far more formidable weapons of attack and defense than the mammals have, and yet they became extinct at about the time the mammalian design was developed in the course of evolution. Mammals are generally more vulnerable than reptiles, but they are also more adaptable. The integrative activity of their brains provides for maintaining the temperature of the blood more or less constant in the face of variations of 100 degrees or more in the surrounding atmosphere. Also, mammals are able to adapt to wetness and dryness, to altitude, and to the wily predatory maneuvers of their enemies. It would appear, therefore, that the purpose of the brain may be not only to maintain constancy of the internal environment, but also to permit effective adaptations to changes in the external environment.

Neural integration is a complex system involving receptor and effector activity and something connecting the two. The connection may be direct, as in a simple reflex arc, or roundabout through interposed neural circuits concerned with interpretation, association with learned experiences, and other stored information either on a conscious or unconscious level. Thus, neural integrative activity refers to what takes place between the delivery of an afferent impulse to the central nervous system and the formation of an efferent pattern of response. It may occur at several levels of the nervous system. When language or other types of symbolism are involved, the process must include the highest integrative level, the cerebral cortex. Thus the ultimate effector pattern may often depend upon the peculiar meaning or significance of a circumstance or event to the particular individual concerned. MacLean has suggested that all afferent information may be available to the hippocampus, an area considered important to affective and visceral behavior (MacLean, 1955–56).

Influx of afferent impulses does not necessarily imply sensation. The viscera provide a profusion of afferent impulses that are not felt but that can be recognized through action potentials picked up from various sub-cortical sites. Both Russian and American workers have picked up a feedback in the brain from simple movements of the stomach (Dunlop, 1958). Such afferents may provide the stimulus for patterning adaptive reactions in disease.

The psychologic interaction of human beings, the relationship of people to each other and to groups may be pathogenic on the one hand or helpful to your health on the other, depending on circumstances. In fact, when the influence of the brain is removed, the general expressions of systemic diseases may be greatly altered. Philip Bard has shown that without the cerebral hemispheres but with the brain stem intact—including the hy-pothalamus—a cat will not react with fever to the injection of a pyro-genic substance (Bard & Woods, 1959). Anaphylactic reactions to powerful antigens have been blocked by anesthesia and, in animals, also by ablation of the tegmentum of the midbrain (Freedman & Fenichel, 1957). Adaptations are accomplished through a rich complex of entero-as well as exteroceptor pathways that subserve interactions or transac-tions between various levels of the central nervous system and other bodily functions, especially the glands of internal secretion. Thus, neural activ-ity may alter thyroid function (Harris & Woods, 1957), for example, and, in turn, variations in the amount of thyroid hormone secreted may have a profound and long-lasting effect on oxygen uptake by the brain (Potapova, 1938).

It has become customary to substitute the terms "input" and "output" for the classical designations "stimulus" and "response." Input informa-tion reaches the highest integrative levels of the nervous system by a variety of routes including the nerves and the blood. The signals may be electrical, mechanical, or chemical, each affecting a specialized type of receptor. If the resulting neural impulse reaches consciousness, it be-comes a sensation. Whether or not sensory information reaches conscious-ness, however, does not necessarily determine the nature or extent of the reaction, or output, except as will, desire, or motivation may add to the picture. Moreover, emotional responses may be aroused, such as fear, anxiety, or resentment, with or without awareness of the original input. Also, with or without awareness, and with or without an emotion or feeling-state, responses may be formulated in terms of striving, creating, destroying, avoiding, and so forth. Thus, frustration of aims and misfortunes may as well lead (and perhaps be essential) to the growth and strengthening of a person as they may to maladaptive reactions. The degree to which energy fed into the organism through afferent channels is essential to his well-being has not as yet been established. Certain it is, however, that a challenge to adapt can promote welfare and productivity. Hans Vaihinger stated, "Man owes his mental development more to his enemies (adversities) than to his friends" (Vaihinger, 1949). The oyster produces the pearl in response to a stress stimulus.

Central Neural Mechanisms and Disease

As W. Grey Walter has put it, "Facts accumulate at a far higher rate than does the understanding of them" (Walter, 1953). So it has been with facts relating the functions of the brain to disease. While vast new knowledge has accumulated concerning the behavior of neurons, of neurotransmitters, receptors, and in the chemistry and physics of neuronal communication in the brain, explanatory information from studies of neurovisceral control continues to be more or less restricted to the activities of autonomic nerves. It has taken a long time for American physicians, and physiologists to move "north" of the brain stem in their inquiries into neural mechanisms of disease. Their focus has favored the hindbrain where the autonomic nerves originate and function mainly as conduits for messages from higher centers in the forebrain where afferent information from within the body and from the environment is perceived, evaluated, and acted upon.

While English-speaking neurophysiologists are now vigorously exploring the forebrain, they are only beginning to formulate their findings regarding intercommunications and interactions in the forebrain in psychological terms. Conversely, as the neuroscientists have uncovered facts relating the functions of the brain to those of the rest of the body, they have had relatively little effect on the thinking of most psychiatrists. Neither have the findings of the neurophysiologists been incorporated into the thinking of most physicians and clinical investigators whose special fields embrace the internal organs, such as the cardiovascular system, the lungs, the kidneys, and so forth.

The Russians are a good deal further along than we are in understanding the relation of the nervous system to disease, thanks to the influence of a contemporary of William Osler named Botkin who, as a teacher and close associate of Pavlov, emphasized the importance of the cerebral cortex to clinical medicine. He evolved a theory of disease based on the work of his compatriot Sechenov and called it "nervism."[2] In it he proposed that most, if not all bodily processes are subject to some sort of regulation by cortical mechanisms—or, in our terms, neural integrative activity.

Sechenov, who had worked under Botkin and Claude Bernard, was impressed not so much by Bernard's constancy of the *milieu interieur* as by its capacity to adapt, presumably under nervous control, to changes in the *milieu exterieur,* and thus protect the organism. Sechenov had probably been influenced by Charles Richet's publication on the "Defense of the Organism" (Richet, 1900). Walter Cannon later credited Richet's work for his concept of Homeostasis (Cannon, 1926). Sechenov had expressed his ideas in a book called *Reflexes of the Brain*, originally published in 1863 and later translated (Sechenov, 1952). It aroused severe criticism from orthodox official tsarist Russia, and became identified with the growth of the philosophy of dialectic materialism and the resultant political changes. In the scientific world, however, Sechenov and his book inspired Pavlov's experimental work and his discovery of the conditional reflex. Since the death of Pavlov, his pupil, Bykov, with a great number of collaborators, accumulated an enormous body of evidence relating efferent and afferent connections of the cerebral cortex to a wide variety of visceral functions, including tissue metabolism (Bykov, 1957).

Symptom Production

Convincing evidence of the power of the nervous system over the rest of the body may be adduced from our everyday experience and without the artifacts of laboratory experimentation. Such is the case when the stimulus is a symbol that has no intrinsic force of its own but that undergoes interpretation by the brain and thereby gains its power. Hearing words that impart good news or bad, seeing a frightening sight, smelling a reminiscent odor, or taking into the mouth a substance with a disgusting taste may provide appropriate input for a variety of complex effector activities in the body. Nausea, with accompanying changes in motor activity of the stomach and duodenum, can be produced not only by emetic drugs and vestibular stimulation, but, by a discussion of pregnancy in the case of a non-pregnant young woman who dreaded the possibility of being pregnant (Wolf, 1955) (figure 6.1). Nausea is always accompanied by interruption of gastric motor activity, loss of gastric tonus, and usually by a transitory increase in the contractile state of the duodenum. In this experiment, the mention of pregnancy was followed by a sudden cessation of vigorous waves of gastric motor activity, a transitory increase in the contractile state of the duodenum, and nausea. This condition might be called hyperemesis gravidarum praecox, because the young woman was not pregnant at the time. The mere discussion of the pregnancy made her ill. A similar experience was that of a hospitalized soldier during the New Guinea campaign in World War II. It was possible to observe, fluoroscopically, complete cessation of gastric movements with accompanying nausea simply by initiating a discussion of lurking Japanese or the horrors of the jungle (Wolf, 1947).

The pain of migraine involves dilatation of arteries in the scalp, supplemented by antidromic transfer of the polypeptide, "neurokinin," to the nerve terminals in the arterial walls. Similarly the pain of inflammation involves a neural transmitter (Chapman et al., 1959). Other evidence that innervation may be implicated in tissue reactivity was adduced by Coburn (1960) in the case of rheumatic nodules and by Smith and associates (Smith et al., 1960) with respect to the experimental production of atrophic gastritis. Flavell found that the mechanisms responsible for hypertrophic pulmonary osteoarthropathy depend upon afferent impulses transmitted from a diseased lung through the vagus nerve to the brain stem (Flavell, 1956). Calvert and Brody adduced evidence that the hepatic damage from carbon tetrachloride is dependent in part on the sympathetic innervation of the liver (Calvert et al., 1960), and the studies of Hampton and associates indicate that the vagus is implicated in the process of fibrin synthesis (Hampton, et al., 1966). These preliminary, but highly provocative, observations on the importance of peripheral nerves to various tissue reactions were reinforced by experiments of Eccles in which the peripheral nerves to the soleus and gastrocnemius were sectioned in the newborn kitten and resutured in reverse (Eccles, 1959). After regeneration Eccles and Buller recorded slow muscle potential from the gastrocnemius (normally fast), and fast waves from the soleus (normally slow) (Buller et al., 1960). Since then, Pette has shown that the characteristics of myocytes are fully under the control of the nervous system (Pette, 1992).

Figure 6.1

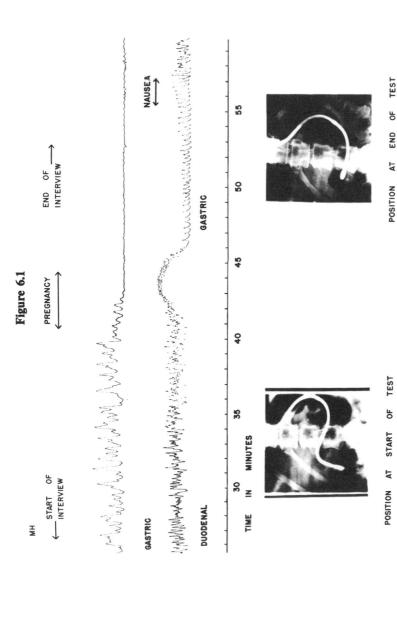

Duodenal spasm with interruption of gastric contractions associated with retrograde movement of the balloon during stressful interview of a young woman discussing possibilities of pregnancy.

Just as neural mechanisms are capable of setting in motion many of the manifestations of disease, so are they capable of mitigating them. The evidence lies in the often efficacious effects of placebo therapy and in the success of a physician in whom the patient has confidence. This idea was expressed by Burton in his *Anatomy of Melancholy*. "An empirick oft times and a silly chirurgeon doth more strange cures than a rational physician...because the patient puts his confidence in him.... He doth the best cures, according to Hippocrates, in whom most trust" (Burton 1891). William Osler recognized this when he said, "It is much more important to know what sort of a patient has a disease than what sort of a disease a patient has" (Osler, 1959).

A great deal of data concerning connections between the viscera and the highest integrative neural centers may be obtained from studies with placebos, which have been used for centuries by physicians under pressure to "do something," but wishing to do no harm. Traditionally, the function of the placebo was to pacify without actually benefiting the patient. The benefit, however, often proves to be unexpectedly lavish. Not only does the hopeful reassurance of placebos engender in patients a feeling of increased well-being, but experimental evidence has shown that placebo administration may be followed by substantial and measurable changes in bodily mechanisms. The objective data to be discussed in chapter 8, are available in published reports and include alterations in pulmonary, gastrointestinal, urogenital, and adrenocortical functions, among others (Wolf, 1959). Therefore, since placebos do a great deal more than placate or pacify, a new definition may be offered as follows: A placebo effect is any effect attributable to a pill, potion, or procedure, but not to its pharmacodynamic or specific properties. Placebo effects derive from the significance to the patient of the whole situation surrounding the therapeutic effort. A connection is thus implied between the particular end organ and the interpretive areas of the brain. Placebo effects may be mediated by autonomic pathways, by other neural channels, or through humoral mechanisms. Relatively few of the routes are really well understood, but it has been shown that virtually all organs and organ systems are capable of responding to stimuli arising out of meaningful situations.

The degree to which disturbances in the environment provoke disease patterns by activating neural structures is incompletely understood. Certainly the various specialized receptors such as baroreceptors, osmoreceptors, and chemoreceptors in blood vessels and in the brain itself are sensitive to minor changes in the composition of the blood, especially to reductions in oxygen tension or alterations in blood pH. In many instances it is known that the nerve impulses activated thereby may result in widespread and often disabling bodily changes (Heymans, 1960). Stimulation by electrodes implanted in the nervous system has produced disturbances in blood coagulation (Gunn & Hampton, 1967), renal function (Hoff et al., 1951) and a variety of endocrine effects including hypertrophy of the thyroid (D'Angelo, 1958). Manning, Hall, and Banting induced myocardial fibrosis in cats and dogs by prolonged stimulation of the vagus (Manning et al., 1937). Gunn and Friedman have shown that lesions in the aorta and coronary arteries of rabbits produced by atherogenic diets can be greatly accentuated by stimulating chronically implanted diencephalic electrodes (Gunn et al., 1968). Lipemia was also significantly greater in the stimulated animals. Seifter and associates have attributed a lipid-mobilizing effect to the pituitary under neural control (Seifter et al., 1959). In our own studies, elevations of serum lipids have been achieved in humans during emotionally charged experiences while the subjects were on a rigidly controlled diet on a metabolic ward (Hammersten et al., 1962).

The processes of renal excretion provides an excellent example of the integrative activity of the central nervous system. Several of the mechanisms that govern the amount and concentration of urine excreted have been shown to be subject to the influence of neural impulses. The evidence in animals was derived from experiments in which parts of the nervous system were stimulated or ablated. In humans, the studies of Schottstaedt and his collaborators are particularly notable (Schottstaedt et al., 1956). They were able to observe a diuresis of sodium and water in healthy subjects on a constant fluid and electrolyte intake under circumstances in which aggressive feelings were aroused. On the other hand, a pronounced retention of both sodium and water occurred in their subjects under circumstances marked by dejection or emotional restraint. The findings were confirmed and found to be of particular significance in a study of patients with borderline congestive heart failure (Barnes & Schottstaedt, 1958).

Other such examples have been encountered in experimental studies on the nose (Holmes et al., 1950), bladder (Straub et al., 1949), esophagus (Wolf & Almy, 1949), colon (Grace et al., 1951), heart (Wolf et al., 1955), and skin (Graham, 1950).

Stress

Stress, for the purpose of discussion, is present when the adaptive mechanisms of the living organism—in this instance, man—are taxed or strained. The widespread acceptance in medicine of the term "stress" has led to the assumption that stress is something specific from which one might anticipate a specific bodily response. On the contrary, a stress is about as specific as an experience since, through the integrative activity of the brain, the event may elicit almost any kind of response—from invention or creation to surrender or death.

Important discoveries, works of art, and advances in thought have been made under the influence of stress. Reaction to stress may thus be measured in terms of achievement, or of the development of fresh potentials—but also in terms of the maintenance of equilibrium or in terms of failure of adaptation, behavior disturbances, and disease. The variety of adaptations is legion and, therefore, the mechanisms subserving them must be similarly numerous.

The Individual and His Disease

The characteristics of an individual are partly inborn and partly acquired. Stimuli encountered in the course of day-to-day living—situations that challenge, threaten, or satisfy—may evoke characteristic patterns of reaction in each individual. The stimulus does not necessarily determine the pattern of response. The determinants include genetic equipment and other characteristics of the individual during development or from experience acquired. Thus, the effect of the stimulus, must depend heavily on the prevailing state of the organism. The pertinence of the stimulus as a determinant of the pattern of response, derives simply from the fact that it is the most recent event. Neither can one explain the phenomena observed in response to a symbolic stimulus in terms of the degree of emotional vulnerability of a particular subject or in terms of nervous imbalance. As obtains with respect to exposure to infectious agents, it can simply be said that some people adapt more smoothly and effectively than others and thus remain healthier.

The proposition that bodily illness may stem more or less directly from neural processes concerned with the formulation and fulfillment of purposes seems appropriate enough and yet difficult to accept fully. The dilemma in the minds of students of disease has been expressed in confused terminology: in the term "psychogenic," for example, and in the meaningless distinction between "organic" and "functional." All diseases are at once functional and organic in the sense that their expression is a disturbance in *function* of some *organ* of the body with or without associated structural change or tissue damage. Thus, the distinction between physical disease and mental disease has little meaning since the brain is an integral part of the human organism.

Reactions in Anticipation

Most people are familiar with the fact that their saliva may flow in anticipation of eating and exercise physiologists are familiar with the increase in cardiovascular activity prior to a race. There are other ways in which the organism may act in anticipation of a stimulus or event. Such anticipatory behavior is a phylogenetically ancient protective adaptation and has been observed in the neural tissue in such lowly forms as sea urchins:

> Because light seems to be somewhat injurious to it, the sea urchin naturally tends to remain in dark places. Yet it responds to a sudden shadow falling upon its body by pointing its spine in the direction from which the shadow comes. This response is defensive, serving to protect the sea urchin from enemies that might have caused the shadow in approaching. The reaction is elicited by the shadow, but it refers to something symbolized by the shadow as is well known. Similar symbolic reactions reach a complex development in higher animals. In man indeed, practically all responses to things seen or heard are merely reactions to representative stimuli. Just as comparative studies in metabolism have revealed a remarkable unity in all the biochemical phenomena of life, so studies of behavior have brought out certain patterns which, formally at least, are common to all living beings. (Dubos, 1959)

Rushmer has observed characteristic changes in left ventricular function in dogs accustomed to treadmill studies merely by showing the animal the treadmill switch (Rushmer & Smith, 1959). In man, a great variety of reactions in anticipation have been studied experimentally. Not only is there tachycardia and increased cardiac output with lowered peripheral resistance in a man preparing for a race, but precisely the same bodily reaction also occurs in the man who his driving is automobile and suddenly hears the shrill sound of motorcycle policeman's siren. He is not running or even planning to run, if he is wise, and yet his cardiovascular apparatus behaves *as if* his muscles needed added nourishment. Such a bodily reaction, "as if," implies that the mechanisms in question are connected with and capable of reacting to impulses from the highest integrative centers of the brain. The biological reaction "as if" occurs most typically in anticipation of some experience—the flow of saliva prior to the mouthing of a tasty morsel or the flow of acid gastric juice in the stomach of a hungry man. It is now equally well recognized that such bodily reactions, "as if," may occur when there is no conscious or obvious connection with the action to which the bodily changes are appropriate. The gastric juice may flow profusely when an individual is frustrated and hostile and quite without appetite.

Theories Relating "As If" to Disease

Essential Hypertension: As If Blood Loss were Threatened

The only uniformly observable bodily change that characterizes essential hypertension is an increase in cardiac output or in peripheral vascular resistance associated with sustained arteriolar constriction. The biological purpose of such a reaction, when imposed upon an initially normal blood pressure, is difficult to perceive. When blood pressure is low, however, as in the shock from blood loss, the pressor response of increased peripheral resistance bolsters what would otherwise be a lagging blood flow throughout the body, and especially in the important areas of the brain and heart. Indeed, hypertension has been induced when cerebral blood flow has been reduced by a variety of means (Guyton, 1948), and years ago Cohnheim proposed that essential hypertension developed as part of an effort of the body to better perfuse the brain (Cohnheim, 1890). It is possible to induce experimentally and predictably an increase in peripheral resistance with an actual elevation of blood pressure during bloodletting from transfusion donors (Wolf, et al., 1955). Indeed, a blood pressure rise attributable to increased peripheral resistance was often encountered prior to the venepuncture and in anticipation of the blood loss. The striking similarity between the hemodynamic adaptive response to bloodletting and the disordered state of essential hypertension may be a matter of coincidence. On the other hand, the hypertensive patient might be viewed as overcompensating for an unconsciously anticipated injury or blood loss. Those who have studied hypertensive patients psychologically have found them poised for aggression yet restraining any aggressive activity and avoiding conflict. An extremely ingenious experimental situation calculated to arouse and yet restrain aggressive impulses was contrived by the Russian workers at the primate laboratory in Zukhumi (Utkin, 1958). Baboons that had self-selected mates were separated. The female was placed in a large cage with a strange male while her mate was placed in a smaller cage alongside. The cuckolded male regularly developed a sustained hypertension. It would be difficult to envision a situation better suited to testing the effects of restrained aggression.

Duodenal Ulcer: Readiness to Devour

Apart from the lesion in the duodenal mucosa, the only bodily change that is known uniformly to accompany peptic ulcer disease is an excessive production of gastric hydrochloric acid and pepsin; excessive because it is sustained rather than intermittent. Each of us at mealtime secretes large amounts of gastric juice with a high concentration of acid and pepsin appropriate to digestion. The gastric behavior of a peptic ulcer patient is *as if* he were always devouring or receiving nourishment. One of the most effective elements in the treatment of the disease is more or less continuous feeding. In the jungle period of man's evolutionary development the appropriate thing to do with an opponent or adversary was to kill and eat him. Thus the linking of gastric hypersecretion of acid and pepsin with circumstances that arouse hostility or resentment may have been a purposeful pattern acquired through mutation. Perhaps the pattern has not been obsolete long enough for civilized man to have lost it through further mutations. It has been observed and repeatedly confirmed that stressful circumstances in the lives of patients with peptic ulcer, especially circumstances that arouse hostile feelings, may be associated with acceleration of the secretion of gastric acid and pepsin. Perhaps it is more than coincidence, therefore, that those who have studied patients with peptic ulcers from a psychological standpoint have found them a lean, hungry, competitive lot.

Diabetes Mellitus: As If One were Starving

The characteristic metabolic change in diabetes mellitus is a tendency to substitute fat for glucose as fuel for metabolic needs. The circumstance under which such a response would be most appropriate is starvation; and indeed, during starvation glucose breakdown is reserved for the nervous tissues and the testes, the only obligatory burners of glucose. The liver makes available the metabolites of fat as a source of energy for the remainder of the body (Keys et al., 1950). For years psychiatrists have pointed out the frequent association of obesity with diabetes and the psychological identification in the minds of diabetic patients of food with love. Juvenile diabetes is most commonly preceded by a period of obesity, and usually there is evidence of deprivation of love during the infantile period (Hinkle, 1951; Daniels, 1939; Dunbar, 1938).

*Coronary Artery Disease: Effort as a Way of Life,
the "Sisyphus" Reaction*

The evidence whereby coronary artery disease is related to an increased serum concentration of cholesterol and lipids is still incomplete. Available data relating lipid mobilization to exercise, however, would indicate that in view of the relatively small amount of glucose available in the body, vigorous muscular activity inevitably requires the mobilization of lipids to satisfy energy needs. The patient with hyperlipemia behaves biologically as if he were undertaking or about to undertake vigorous effort. In the light of this it is striking that four groups of investigators who have reported psychological studies of patients with coronary artery disease find them to be distinctly effort-oriented (Groover, 1957; Hammersten et al., 1957; Russek & Zohman, 1958; Friedman & Rosenman, 1959). In our own studies we found these patients to have a strong desire to do things on their own. They felt a great need to be responsible for what they did and delegated authority with difficulty. Moreover, they showed very little tendency to rest between labors; instead of savoring the satisfactions of accomplishment, they went on to meet the next challenge. This suggested designating theirs the "Sisyphus" pattern since Sisyphus, when confined in Hades, was required to push a great rock up a steep hill; whenever he was near the top, the rock rolled down again and required that he continue the effort.

Modern man is inclined to encounter noxious stimuli, or stresses of a symbolic nature, far more frequently than directly damaging assaults. His responses, which, as we have seen, may involve his whole being in the direction of health or disease, depend upon his goals and values. Thus they constitute his way of life. Throughout man's evolution, the quality of his performance has reflected the validity of his values. In terms of social as well as bodily health, he has often been more unadapted than adapted, more sick than well.

Among the adaptations required in Western civilization are many age-old ones and certain characteristically modern ones, including those inherent in a fluid social class structure. Other important factors are the conflict between Old World cultural pressures and those encountered in the United States as well as problems arising from instabilities in the family structure (Wolff, 1953). The body may respond with disease patterns not only to tangible noxae, but just as readily to stimuli that owe their force not to their intrinsic qualities but to their meaning to the individual. Cultural and social pressures share with universal psychological drives and inborn personal proclivities the ability to shape or modify the interpretation of experience and thereby bear upon the character of the bodily response that results. Thereby is formed the basis of a connection between the social sciences and medicine.

Essentially, it appears that man needs to live in a fashion acceptable to his fellows. He needs to derive spiritual nourishment from his activities and the things that happen to him, and he needs to satisfy in some way his various emotional needs and to realize his potential for love and for creativity. Threats to his ability to perform in all of these spheres constitute the important everyday stresses that are apparently behind so many states of disability and disease. A preventive emphasis in medicine demands that we take into consideration all of these factors and that we attempt to develop satisfactory ways of dealing with them individually and collectively.

We are gradually learning that in biology the only permanent thing is change—change requiring ever new adaptive responses on the part of organisms, races, and species to serve their need to survive. Man's thinking brain has both aided him in his adaptations and created new challenges for him. His science and technology have provided protection from the elements and from other destructive forces in the environment. They have also confronted him with new hazards of injury, accidental death, and subtler changes as well in the form of radiations and noxious chemicals in the air he breathes and in the food he eats. Man's reckless and apparently insatiable desire to explore and experiment has led him to establish a kind of mastery over the world despite his diminutive stature, the delicacy of his offspring, and his lack of natural weapons such as sharp teeth or claws.

Disability and death resulting from exposure to the elements were mitigated when man sought shelter and clothing; then the wild predators were fended off with arms and the microbes with public hygiene and antibiotics. Now the illnesses related to man's own productions and his relations with his fellow man are gaining prominence. The creation of societies required that males learn to live together without destroying each other; now the survival of society requires that we learn to tolerate differences in people and their points of view. The stresses concerned with this step in development provide much of what is noxious in the environment of modern man. These forces combine with others that tradition has already acknowledged to limit him through disability and discomfort. It is with relevant and potentially relevant factors, then, that we must concern ourselves in examining disease mechanisms. Taking due cognizance of genetic proclivities, learned patterns of response, and pressures of all sorts—tangible and otherwise—we must look for the forces that arouse and the mechanisms that modulate adaptive efforts in the body. This means that we must abandon the search for the will-o'-the-wisp, the single ultimate cause, and see man's state of being—his health or illness—as an aspect of his way of life.[3]

Notes

1. René Dubos, professor of environmental medicine at Rockefeller Institute and University for fifty years, discovered gramicidin, the first antibiotic from soil bacteria. He was an intellectual leader among medical scientists and wrote several books on the interrelationship between social forces, personal development, and disease.
2. Sergei Petrovich Botkin (1832–1889), who was born seventeen years before Osler, played a role in Russian medicine that was very similar to that of Osler in the English-speaking countries. A broadly educated, deeply committed bedside physician and teacher, Botkin was a strong advocate and stimulator of clinical research. His theory of nervism stated that all bodily processes are regulated by the central nervous system (Brazier, 1959).
3. The persistence of those who hold the genes responsible for most major diseases is based on the assumption that genes from several chromosomes combine to provide the underlying pathological mechanisms. Genetic proclivity may be a factor in the causation of numerous diseases but only a small number of diseases (perhaps 2 percent) can be thought of as genetically determined. Nevertheless the possibility of molecular genetics being capable of explaining the cause and mechanism many of the major diseases of the present era has captured the attention of the medical research community despite considerable evidence to the contrary (Strohman, 1995).

7

From Information to Understanding: The Challenge for the Library

"Information, like entertainment, is something someone else provides us. Each of us must acquire knowledge for ourself. Knowledge comes from the free mind foraging in rich pasture of the whole everywhere past."

—Daniel Boorstin, director,
Library of Congress

An important characteristic of human beings is that they have no genetic mechanism for passing on learning from one generation to another. This means, of course, that every new-born human must start from scratch vis-à-vis the accumulated fund of knowledge. Here lies the significance of the library, to preserve and communicate learning, and, as an increasingly important function, to organize it. William Osler likened efforts to learn medicine without a library to sailing a ship without a tiller. On the other hand, he compared relying on the library without hands-on experience with patients to a ship remaining stationary (Osler, 1903).

History

As did so much of our ancient heritage, libraries began in Mesopotamia where the Sumerians etched cuneiform figures into clay tablets and stored them in shelters. Such storehouses, probably established around the twenty-first century B.C., could be thought of as the first libraries. Other ancient libraries were established in Assyria, Babylonia, Egypt, Greece, Jerusalem, Alexandria, Pergamum, and Rome during the succeeding centuries. They were originally used to preserve commercial documents, but later became store houses for knowledge concerning religious and political matters.

The first library opened for study by learned scholars was probably the one founded in Alexandria in the first century B.C. during the rule of Ptolomy I. This magnificent resource of civilization was destroyed in the year 391 A.D. by the Roman emperor Theodocius I who was carrying out a campaign against pagan institutions.[1] The most distinguished library still in existence at that time was the one built in Nineveh by the Assyrians in the mid-seventh century B.C. Long after it too was destroyed, the ever-present British archaeologists gathered up its cuneiform tablets and brought them to the British museum in London where they are still to be seen.

After clay tablets, writings were preserved on scrolls made of Egyptian papyrus until paper was invented in China. News of this discovery did not reach Europe until the Chinese war with the Arabs at Samarkand in 751 A.D. The Arabs lost the war but went away knowing how to make paper. The Christian monks laboriously copied the Bible, other sacred documents, and Gregorian chants on parchment. They decorated the first letter of each chapter with gold leaf. Later, in the twelfth century, the knowledge of paper filtered into Europe. A few hundred years after that there followed the reinvention of printing, another innovation that had appeared in the Orient long before. Libraries were scattered throughout the known world during the Renaissance.

The Working Library

As information accumulated and knowledge grew, it became necessary for libraries to devise ways of organizing the growing mass of data and opinion in order to make it available to the reader. A series of innovations in searching and cataloging followed, most of them adapted to the concept of the library as curator of knowledge.

Until recently, most librarians enjoyed a quiet, contemplative but busy life. The stereotype of the library was a quiet room where voices must be hushed or even silent, virtually eliminating most verbal communication. The librarian was depicted as a sharp-eyed guardian of the collection who possessed an uncanny ability to locate an obscure quote or a forgotten reference.

Times have changed! While libraries and librarians, with their impressive technical resources, continue to engage in their hording and locating functions, they have assumed a vital role in the processes of educational information and communication.

Communication Among Libraries

It is hard to identify where or when the working library started, but it may be possible to credit Gottfried von Leibniz, the great seventeenth-century philosopher and mathematician, who focused on the importance of bibliographic research and communication among scholars. It is interesting that Leibniz perfected Blaise Pascal's adding machine and thereby began the portentous development of the calculating machine, which, with the approach of the computer age, was to exert such an enormous influence on our lives.

In 1786 the American Library Association was founded. Its initial great contribution was to promote free access to materials, not just in one library, but in any library. Interlibrary cooperation, the development of the intensive searches and loans, was a bright chapter in American history. One of the founders of the American Library Association, Melville Dewey (not to be confused with John Dewey), proposed the decimal system for classification in 1876. A few years later, Charles Richet, professor of physiology at the University of Paris, was working toward the same goal. He dropped his scheme when he learned of the Dewey Decimal System being used in the U.S. Richet then turned his efforts toward developing a compendium of knowledge of physiology from the beginning of recorded history. This multiple authored encyclopedia, the *Dictionnaire de Physiologie*, was started in 1895 with the letter A. Each year a new volume appeared until the operation was interrupted by World War I. The last volume was published in 1913. Unfortunately, the work had reached only to the L's. The last page of the last volume contains a photograph of the first volume lighted up by luminescent organisms, thereby illustrating the last subject, LU, biological luminescence.

Richet's extraordinary achievement was something that current mechanized devices are failing to do. With their extraordinary speed of responsiveness, they are failing to provide an historical perspective for scientific progress. In fact, there is so little emphasis on the history of discovery that we now find ourselves in an era where crucial observations and concepts are being rediscovered. They are being rediscovered because busy investigators, under pressure to produce papers, are only going back a few years in their literature search, only as far as the new mechanized services can reach back. The occurrance of this uncivil behavior is the not uncommon. Rediscovery of phenomena that had already been described in the literature continues to occur. It will happen more and more frequently as we continue to assign time saving self-celebration as the highest priority.

The Active Library

The active library is characterized by intensification of interlibrary cooperation and communication as well as by rapidly advancing bibliographic and other skilled personal and computerized services. Medical libraries have contributed substantially to this development.[2] *The Index Medicus, Medlars,* and their several computerized progeny, as well as other reference programs developed over the past twenty years, have defined the active library. It evolved without sacrificing its more traditional organized archival functions. The National Library of Medicine, by the use of satellite communication reaches doctors and hospitals in remote places with needed information. By virtue of its extramural programs, its funding of critical reviews and its support of scholarly work and publications, the library is projecting itself into the community of scholars, physicians, and scientists world wide.

A New Challenge, Synthesis

The mission of the library is to support scholarship by better organizing the products of learning and making them more readily available. There remains a pressing need on the part of practicing physicians and medical scientists alike for synthesis of an increasing mass of information pouring into libraries from many disciplines and specialized areas of study concerned with human health and disease.

The difficulty of such a task is accentuated by the growing tendency of medical scientists to partition their activities and interests into rapidly proliferating specialty meetings and journals that tend to isolate the disciplines from one another. Unfortunately, their specialized languages are almost as disparate as those of the builders of the Tower of Babel. Thus the rapid progress of research in several areas basic to medicine, including the behavioral sciences, has created a challenging paradox—specialization with ever-narrowing interests of investigators in the face of an increasing need for medical students, researchers, and practitioners to gain a broad understanding of man and his world.

Since new data turned up in one field of study might find application in another, intercommunication among disciplines is needed, but has been impeded by the isolation of specialties. Hence vision is obstructed by a lush growth of technical esoterica in the language of each special field. The more highly specialized biological research has become, the greater has been the difficulty of appreciating the applications of its discoveries. Not only are we discovering more, but we are unable to put together what has been discovered. As a consequence, we have been faced with a series—almost a jumble—of rapidly moving frontiers that cry out for connections and conceptual definition.

Perhaps the next step for medical libraries should be to develop techniques and strategies to help make the rapidly proliferating mass of information not only accessible, but intelligible. It may, be important for libraries to encourage the publication of interdisciplinary discourse, carried out in such a way that the findings in one field can be understood in terms of the needs and concepts of another.

One promising effort in this direction was attempted in a conference on arteriosclerosis held in the spring of 1970. It was convened because arteriosclerosis, a multifaceted disorder so important to Western society, had attracted researchers from several more or less separate basic and clinical disciplines. Each group of investigators was approaching the problem with its own special techniques, conceptions, and language. The conference was held at Lindau on Lake Constance in Germany. It brought together 122 individuals from twenty countries for a colloquium that lasted five and a half days. Throughout that period there were only six formal presentations, each lasting forty-five minutes. Most of the time was spent in discussion guided by very skillful chairmen who encouraged communication among the scientists of varied background representing a wide range of biomedical disciplines. The chairmen tried to translate the in-group jargon in each area of study and thereby to mitigate the natural embarrassment of individuals who, unfamiliar with the technology of a certain area, hesitated to speak. The chairmen not only encouraged participation but even called on those who had something to offer but were reluctant to speak. Thus, biochemists, pathologists, neurobiologists, the entire gamut of individuals from the differing disciplines, were learning to talk to each other. It seemed like a step toward correcting the problem of the Tower of Babel (Wolf, 1971).

Among the accomplishments of the conference was a partial reconciliation of seven apparently mutually exclusive theories of the pathogenesis of arteriosclerosis. After five and a half days of discussion nearly everyone left with a sense of broadened and deepened understanding and new ideas to use in future inquiry.[3]

The lessons from this effort of synthesis have subsequently been applied to ten smaller additional colloquia with approximately thirty participants. Each one was sponsored by the Totts Gap Institute in Bangor, Pennsylvania. They dealt with the following topics: Smooth Muscle of the Artery, The Biology of the Schizophrenic Process, The Limits of Medicine: The Doctor's Job in the Coming Era, The Dynamics of Arterial Flow, The Technological Imperative in Medicine, The Composition and Function of Cell Membranes, Structure and Function of the Circulation, Genetic Analysis of the X Chromosome, Gene Expression in Muscle, and Clinical Trials in Neuromuscular Diseases.

A considerable degree of synthesis emerged from these gatherings. Especially notable among the participants at the colloquia were subsequent collaborations as well as exchanges of graduate and postdoctoral students among investigators who had never met before and often were unaware of each other's publications.

The support of similar colloquia designed to promote scientific synthesis might well become an important role for the library. Such an activity would widen the mainstream of traditional library activity, not by producing new information, but by enhancing its role as a curator of knowledge. By achieving disciplinary intercommunication and synthesis of findings, the library would ultimately serve to advance knowledge.

Notes

1. Theodocius I (347–395 A.D.) ruled the eastern unit of the Roman Empire from 379–395. He was the first Roman emperor to dispense with the pagan title, Pontifix Maximus, and insisted that everyone in the realm be Christian and subscribe to the dogmas of Nicea. He engaged in much cruel suppression, and in 390 was required by St. Ambrose to do public penance for his cruelty. The following year he renewed his attacks on paganism and destroyed the great library at Alexandria.

2. Among the major contributors has been the National Library of Medicine. Dr. Martin M. Cummings, director from 1964–1984, made highly important innovations with computer technology that enabled a physician to make a search of the medical literature from his office. Special rapid search arrangements were made for emergency situations involving drug toxicity, and so on. He built collaborative relationships with major libraries in Europe, Australia, and elsewhere that enriched collections and simplified access to them all over the world. In addition, he arranged for English translation of foreign publications in several languages.

3. The colloquium was held under the auspices of the International Society of Cardiology, the International Cardiology Foundation and the European Atherosclerosis Group. Arrangements for the meeting were directed by Professor Gothard Schettler and Dr. Gunter Schlierf of the University of Heidelberg.

8

The Evaluation of Therapy in Disease

"The young practitioner may bear in mind that patients are more often damaged than helped by the promiscuous drugging which is still only too prevalent." These were the words of Sir William Osler in the introduction to the fifth edition of his textbook of medicine (Osler, 1920). Dr. Eugene DuBois, in his presidential address to the Association of American Physicians, quoted Osler's remarks but further pointed out that Osler, after giving his admonition, went on in the body of his book to recommend for the therapy of pneumonia "bleeding, veratrum viride, Paquelin cautery, hot poultices, cold baths, Dover's powers, and strychnine" (DuBois, 1937). None of these agents would be expected to exert a significant effect on a patient suffering from pneumonia.

The history of therapeutics in medicine, is a troubled one. Among available useful therapeutic agents before World War II were quinine for malaria, the number one killer in the world, salvarsan for syphilis, sulfanilamide for some other infections, aspirin, which was of some benefit in rheumatic fever, digitalis for heart failure, morphine and codeine to relieve suffering, insulin for diabetes, nicotinic acid for pellagra, thiamin for beri beri, and vitamin B_{12} for pernicious anemia plus very few other safe and effective agents.

Since the availability of penicillin after World War II, there has been an enormous proliferation of pharmacological agents designed either to remove the cause, to interfere with the mechanisms, or to relieve the pain and suffering of disease. Today, the pharmaceutical companies of America offer more than 3,000 separate medications. Their products have relieved much suffering, cured some diseases and prolonged many lives. On the other hand, the careless or promiscuous use of pharmaceuticals has too often been harmful.

Hazards and "Side Effects" of Pharmacological Therapy

In the early 1960s Leighton Cluff, a professor of medicine at Johns Hopkins, observed that over the period of one month 10 percent of patients on the medical service had been admitted because of toxic reactions from prescribed medications. More startling was his discovery that 10 percent of the other patients on the wards had, during their hospitalization, acquired toxic reactions from medications prescribed by the staff. Today, despite stringent requirements for efficacy and safety of drugs imposed by the federal government before they can be prescribed, toxic side effects of pharmaceuticals are still frequently encountered.

The continuing hazards of what William Osler called "promiscuous drugging" have been documented by Steel who found that 36 percent of patients admitted to a university medical service in a teaching hospital suffered an iatrogenic event, of which 25 percent were serious or life threatening. More than half of the injuries were related to use of medications (Steel, 1981). In 1991 Bedell et al. (1991) reported the results of an analysis of cardiac arrests at a teaching hospital. They found that 64 percent were preventable. Again, inappropriate use of drugs was the leading cause of the cardiac arrests.

Whether or not the error rates reported above exceed the norm is not known. In any case the authors suggested that treatment errors, when they occur, be shared with the patient, professional colleagues, and the administration of the hospital so that they may be understood and usually forgiven. Such treatment would also facilitate the development of new efforts at error prevention among the staff.

The reasons for errors are legion but the lack of adequately deliberate and thoughtful behavior at the bedside is probably the leading cause. Sometimes hurried phone calls or messages delivered by a surrogate may cause errors in the medications administered. Such short cuts are no substitute for meticulous care.

A further problem has been the failure of the physician to expose the error. The temptation to cover up may stem from an expectation of infallibility by the physician himself, his patient, or his superiors, or from the physician's need to avoid embarrassment or even a malpractice suit. Such cover up behavior, of course, reflects the character of the physician and questions the existing criteria for admission to medical school discussed in chapter 1.

In considering the possible effects of drugs on bodily mechanisms, it is important to bear in mind what other forces might oppose or reinforce their pharmacological action. Apart from the influence of age, sex, attitude, climate, or the presence of other physiological disorders, a clearly relevant factor is the mental and emotional state of the patient.

On one occasion 10cc of syrup of ipecac were administered blindly through an intragastric tube to a pregnant woman who was subject to morning nausea. She was not nauseated at the time and the lack of nausea was documented by the presence of vigorous waves of motor activity which were being recorded from the stomach. Within seven minutes the gastric motor activity stopped abruptly and nausea ensued. A later experiment performed was in the same fashion at a time when the patient was nauseated, and gastric activity was absent. The ipecac was again introduced blindly through the open lumen of the intragastric tube as before, but the patient had been told that she was receiving a new medicine, just imported from Germany, that was sure to correct her troublesome nausea and vomiting. Despite her having received the same dose of ipecac, nausea disappeared within fifteen minutes and gastric motor activity resumed. Had it not been for the recorded tracing of gastric motor activity, one might have assumed that the patient had imagined the disappearance of nausea, but the resumption of gastric motor activity established reliably that there was no longer any nausea.

From these observations it is evident that the effect of a drug may vary from person to person and from time to time in the same person irrespective of the pharmacodynamic properties of the agent in question, depending on the circumstances at the time of the administration. The proof of this inference would be available if there were human subjects whose responses were normal except for an inability to interpret their surroundings. Fortunately, we had the opportunity to study one such subject who had been rendered effectively decorticate in an automobile accident. A study of this individual has been published elsewhere (Doig et al., 1953). Suffice it to say here that he gave no evidence of awareness or responsiveness to his environment but he did display a consistent sleep and awake cycle with eyes closed at night and open during the day. A gastrostomy, which had been done to facilitate his management, offered a convenient opportunity for the study of gastric function. Like our earlier fistulous subject, Tom, this individual displayed cyclic activity in his stomach with periods of accelerated acid secretion every few hours. Accordingly, he was given a small dose (0.4 mgm) of atropine hypodermically at various stages in the cycle of spontaneous gastric activity. A larger dose (0.6 mgm) administered to our subject, Tom, with a long-standing gastric fistula, on one occasion had produced effective inhibition, but on another occasion when Tom was under considerable emotional stress, the atropine caused no gastric inhibition (Wolff & Wolf, 1947). In the "decorticate" subject, however, the smaller dose of atropine was followed uniformally by an inhibitory effect regardless of the prevailing level of secretion.

Design of a Therapeutic Trial

Assuming that a proposed pharmacodynamic agent has been shown to be sufficiently free of toxicity to satisfy the Federal Drug Administration, there are several requirements for a therapeutic trial in order to demonstrate efficacy in the treatment of a particular clinical disorder: (1) it is necessary to show that the sought for change would not have occurred spontaneously; (2) the potential interfering circumstances during the trial must be known and controlled; (3) criteria for a favorable result must be identified and, if possible, measured; (4) the homogeneity with respect to the severity of the disorder of the subjects to be treated must be known and the analysis must be carried out accordingly.

When isoniazid (INH, Nydrazid, Ramifon) was first tried in tuberculosis, patients were photographed dancing in the hospital corridors. Since the drug could not have cured the disease in this length of time, it was concluded that it was exerting a euphorogenic effect. Patients are no longer dancing, and it is now clear that isoniazid is useful in treating tuberculosis but it does not induce euphoria (Miracle Drugs, 1953).[1] The early patients who received the drug were euphoric without a doubt, but the euphoria was not due to the pharmacodynamic properties of the drug. It was probably due to the fact that the physicians of these patients in the tuberculosis hospitals had just been suddenly converted from jailers to therapists, and it was their renewed hope, faith, and pleasure in this event that had rubbed off on the patients and produced euphoria.

Long before systematic methods were developed to test the effects of medications, Pinel had suggested that the therapeutic efficacy of drugs could be tested by treating patients one year and not the next (Pinel, 1803), but his data were not reliable because the severity of disease, especially infectious diseases, varies greatly from year to year. It was failure to recognize this fact that led to the conviction in the minds of many medical leaders in the late 1940s that chlortetracycline (aureomycin) was effective in the treatment of atypical pneumonia (Finland et al., 1949; Kneeland et al., 1949; Meiklejohn, 1949; Olshaker ct al., 1949; Schoenbach, 1949; Woodward, 1949). It was not until four years later (in 1953) and after many hundred of pounds of aureomycin had been used in the treatment of atypical pneumonia that Walker published his controlled study of 212 cases in which aureomycin was found to be no more effective than a placebo (Walker, 1953).

"Take care of the experimental design and the tests of significance will take care of themselves" (Reid, 1954). Attempts to evaluate the efficacy of a treatment by comparing the results of an untreated group with a series treated with a certain therapeutic agent, have failed to bear fruit in one disease after another. For example, Jordan and Kiefer reported in 1932 a series of 392 patients with peptic ulcer treated with a new drug. They documented only a 9 percent recurrence of duodenal ulcer in one year and 46 percent in five years (Jordan & Kiefer, 1932). Emery and Monroe, on the other hand, with an even larger series, reported figures that bore very little resemblance to those of Jordan and Kiefer: 59 percent recurrences in one year and 93 percent in five years (Emery & Monroe, 1935).

With respect to tranquilizing drugs, an experiment was particularly revealing (Feldman, 1956). Their effectiveness was measured by the patients' assessment of how well they had done on each individual tranquilizing drug. In addition, an estimate was made of the degree of enthusiasm that the doctor had for each of the agents. The correlation showed that those patients that had done the best were in the group treated by the doctors who liked the drug best. Those who did poorly were patients of the therapeutic nihilists.

During a study of the effect of heparin on angina pectoris, Janet Travel found that the concentration of lipoproteins in the blood was significantly reduced by heparin and also by blindly administered placebos (figure 8.1). (Rinzler et al., 1953). In another experiment involving fifty-two observations in twenty-six individuals, the incidence of nausea was 100 percent, and of vomiting 85 percent following the oral administration of 6 ml of ipecac. A week later the experiment was repeated with the same group of subjects, but prior to the ipecac an "an-

Figure 8.1

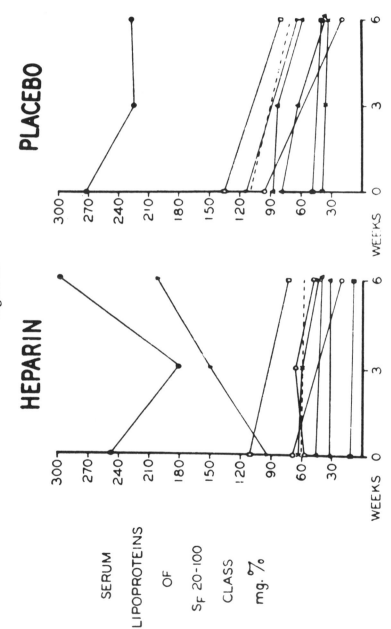

Similar effects of Heparin and Placebo in reducing the concentration of lipoproteins in the blood of human subjects with coronary heart disease.

tiemetic" capsule was administered blindly and randomly to each of them. One-third of the capsules contained chlorpromazine 20 mg, another third Phenothiazine and the other third was a placebo. On this occasion nausea and vomiting were reduced by 20 percent among the subjects taking each of the three agents. Success or failure in the attempt to prevent nausea and vomiting was almost identical for the three different capsules. That is to say that the placebo did just as well or as poorly in preventing nausea and vomiting as did the other two "antiemetics" unknown to the subjects. Had this been an uncontrolled therapeutic trial the 50 to 65 percent "satisfactory" protection against nausea and vomiting afforded by these agents would have been considered clinically significant at the level of $p=0.01$ or less. Only the inclusion of the placebo data prevented the erroneous conclusion that a specific pharmacodynamic effect had been demonstrated.

The Pharmacology of Placebos

The heading presents a picturesque contradiction. Pharmacology concerns itself with the chemical properties of drugs and their effects on biological mechanisms. Placebos produce effects on biological mechanisms independently of their chemical properties. The term "placebo" derives from the Latin "I will please," or "placate." The origins and usages of the term have been elegantly researched and described by Pepper (Pepper, 1945) in a delightful and informative commentary of a sort so rarely offered in present-day medical literature.

Placebos have been used for centuries by physicians under pressure to "do something," but wishing to do no harm. Traditionally, the function of the placebo was to pacify without actually benefiting the patient. The benefit, however, has proved to be unexpectedly lavish. Not only has the hopeful reassurance of placebos engendered in patients a feeling of increased well-being, but experimental evidence has shown that placebo administration may be followed by substantial and measurable changes in bodily mechanisms (Wolf, 1950). Therefore, since placebos do a great deal more than placate or pacify, a new definition may be offered as follows: *Placebo effect = any effect attributable to a pill, potion, or procedure, but not to its pharmacodynamic or specific properties.* Placebo effects derive from the significance to the patient of the whole situation surrounding the therapeutic effort. Thereby is implied a connection between a particular end organ and the interpretive areas of the brain. Placebo effects may be mediated via autonomic pathways, other neural channels, or through humoral mechanisms. Relatively few of the routes are really well understood but certain it is that virtually all organs and organ systems are capable of responding to meaningful situations and among them the administration of placebos.

Historical Perspective

Placebos have been used to alleviate human suffering since the beginnings of medicine, but not usually knowingly. Each medical era has brought forward chemical agents, efficacious at the time, but later found to lack the pertinent pharmacodynamic property. Countless herbs and potions have filled the pages of textbooks as prevailing fashions have changed with each generation, the placebo action of the agents having derived in part from the faith and enthusiasm of earnest physicians. Many such agents have died out reluctantly. When, from time to time, various ones of them have been exposed as chemically useless, new, often more expensive but equally intrinsically inert nostrums have taken their places, each enjoying its day of clinical effectiveness. The placebo acquired a special dignity when, in 1946, it became the subject of one of the Cornell Conferences on Therapy (Wolff, et al., 1946). Harry Gold, who organized the conference, had the perspicacity to take seriously the power of the heretofore humble placebo. He and Garb and their associates had identified various physiological alterations attributable to the placebo (Gold, 1950). Wolff at this same conference told of observed effects of placebos on pain perception (Wolff, et al., 1946). The first evidence of a placebo effect that was documented by measurement of physiological changes in the organ affected was obtained during the studies of Tom, a patient with a gastric fistula (Wolf, 1950).[2]

Modell wrote (Modell, 1958) that the placebo effect "is the only single action which all drugs have in common and in some instances it is the only useful action which the medication can exert." An engaging and articulate tribute to the placebo is contained in the article, already referred to, by Perry Pepper (Pepper, 1955).

Eugene DuBois, in his presidential address to the Association of American Physicians listed three classes of placebos (DuBois, 1939). The first included simple substances, inert and unpretentious, such as lactose and starch. The second class included pseudomedicaments, extracts of herbs, poisonous metals, superfluous vitamins, and so forth. Such are the ingredients of most proprietary medicines sold over the counter. The third is the placebo effect that goes along with the pharmacodynamic action of a specific therapeutic agent (Wolff, et al., 1946).

Among the powerful circumstances that aid the placebo in alleviating symptoms and curing disease is the inherent recuperative power of the human organism, the tendency for diseases to be self-limited. As long ago as 1800, Gall (Gall, 1800) was asking himself, "What is nature's share and what is medicine's in the healing of disease." Before his time, the dictates of authority had determined pretty well what treatments would be used, and the weight of authority was considered adequate as evidence for the efficacy of a particular agent or procedure. Sixty-three years after Gall, bleeding, still honored by authority, was the most popular treatment for pneumonia when Béclard, in one of the first well-controlled therapeutic experiments, proved that bleeding had no specific value (Béclard, 1863). Unsupported inferences concerning medical treatment were widely and easily accepted among the best in the profession. For example, Edward Trudeau had gone up to his favorite haunt in the Adirondack Mountains to die of tuberculosis. When, instead, he recovered, he attributed his conquest of tuberculosis to the mountain air (Trudeau, 1916) and thereby fostered a placebo ritual that long outlived him. He might, with equal justification, have credited the nourishing qualities of the rabbits he shot on the hillside.

The Meaningful Situation

One vivid example of the power of a meaningful situation to bring about striking bodily effects was provided by a woman who had a gastric ulcer. Although her symptoms were typical enough, we were naturally concerned lest her lesion be malignant, particularly because on two occasions she had failed to produce an acid response to histamine (Histamine Phosphate, U.S.P.) This woman had lived an emotionally arid life with many frustrations and few satisfactions. Life with her first husband was as unsatisfactory as it had been with her parents. Ultimately, she divorced this man and somewhat later, met and married a gentle, kind person. He was interesting and interested in her. Her life was soon filled with newfound satisfactions. Things went well until she happened to discover her fine new husband molesting her twelve-year-old daughter by her first husband. If he had robbed a bank, killed his mother, or sold secrets to the Russians, she could probably have gone on living happily with him, standing by him and deriving the satisfactions this marriage afforded, but he had done the one thing that was beyond the pale. At this time, she developed her first symptoms of ulcer. Shortly thereafter, her husband was drafted and sent overseas leaving her in conflict as to what to do. Before he returned, she made the decision not to take him back. On the third occasion of gastric analysis, instead of giving this patient an injection of histamine, she was simply asked, "Tell me why it was that you did not take your husband back when he returned from overseas?" This question, a powerful and meaningful stimulus, was followed by a prompt secretion of gastric acid to 40 mEq/1 when histamine, the most powerful secretory drug available, had failed (Wolf, 1957). From this experience, it is evident that meaningful situations that do not involve the taking of medicaments may equally well affect the organs and organ systems of the human body. This principle is the foundation of psychosomatic medicine. This important fact has soaked only slowly into the scientific consciousness of today and explains the responsiveness of any organ or organ system to placebo therapy. Although less reliable, placebo effects may be as potent as those of well-established agents, as helpful, for example to the patient with rheumatoid arthritis as salicylates or even cortisone (Traut & Passarelli, 1957), as potent in lowering blood pressure as reserpine (Reserpoid, Serpasil) (Palmer, 1955), as useful as opiates in dealing with anguish of the postoperative state (Beecher, 1956). Lasagna and associates showed that several customarily relied upon characteristics of pharmacodynamic agents, including the dose-response curve with "peak" effect, cumulative action, and holdover effects, could be observed during the course of placebo therapy (Lasagna, 1958).

Predictability

Except in the case of a patient's special need, a physician's special hope, or an experimenter's deliberate manipulation of the situation by suggestion, or otherwise, there appears to be nothing predictable about placebo effects. Placebos may induce in an organ a change in one direction or in another, or no change at all. A vivid example of the way a placebo may produce changes in opposite directions in a single organ was described in chapter 2.

Toxic Effects of Placebos

Several authors have observed toxic reactions in response to the administration of placebos (Ewing & Haizlip, 1958; Gravenstein, 1956; Gravenstein, et al., 1956). Sheldon, in a study of reserpine administered to hypertensive patients, found that the patients who were receiving placebos complained of nasal stuffiness as often as did those who were getting reserpine (Sheldon, personal communication). Shapiro and Grollman, studying effects of antihypertensive agents given by mouth to ambulatory patients, found that one of their most troublesome and persistent "Hydralazine" (Apresoline, 1-hydrazinophthalazine hydrochloride) headaches occurred in an individual who was getting placebo at the time (Shapiro & Grollman, 1953). Our own experiences with the toxic effect of placebos included a study of the purported anxiety-relieving effects of the relaxant drug, mephenesin (Tolserol, 3-o-toloxy-1,2 propranediol) (Wolf & Pinsky, 1954). Because it was so difficult to quantify subjective and objective signs of anxiety, five unknown medications were used. Some of them contained the agent and some the placebo. The lack of precision in quantifying the data was thus equalized among the five groups. When the key was finally broken, it was found that the results with the drug and placebo were almost identical (Wolf & Pinsky, 1954). Many of the patients noted minor toxic effects including sleepiness, sleeplessness, anorexia, nausea, tremulousness, dizziness, and palpitation. The incidence of these minor side effects was identical with the placebo and the agent. Three patients had serious toxic reactions. One developed what the dermatologist called "dermatitis medicamentosa" while taking only a placebo. Another individual suddenly collapsed in an anaphylactoid reaction with nausea and lowering of blood pressure, clammy white skin and fainting within fifteen minutes after taking the medication. Identical reactions occurred following the placebo and the agent. The third severe reaction included epigastric pain coming on within ten minutes of taking the pill. This response occurred on three separate occasions with three different batches of pills. Watery diarrhea, urticaria, and angioneurotic edema of the lips followed on each occasion. It later developed that these reactions had occurred first on placebo and then on the drug. Diehl and his associates demonstrated that placebos were as effective as cold vaccines in stopping colds and found also that these placebos were associated with numerous toxic symptoms including drowsiness, lassitude, listlessness, dizziness, giddiness, vertigo, headaches, depression, insomnia, and gastrointestinal disturbances (Diehl, 1933; Diehl et al., 1940). Leslie reported that among morphine addicts in whom saline had been substituted for the drug no withdrawal symptoms were experienced by any of them until the saline injections were stopped (Leslie, 1954). Careful experiments have shown that measurable and often major changes in visceral function may be induced by the situation surrounding the giving of a placebo (Wolf, 1950). For example, a change in the number of circulating eosinophiles has been induced either during discussion of stressful topics or following the administration of placebos (Holmes et al., 1950; Hinkle et al., 1950).

The Mechanisms of Placebo Action

Every contact with a physician may be a meaningful situation to the patient, and hence may set off visceral responses which can have a salutary or adverse effect on health and well being. The same goes for every procedure including surgery and every medicine prescribed. Similarly, the effects of bread pills or any inert placebo are not imaginary but very real.

The stimulus responsible for placebo effects is the meaningful situation. Its force, often underestimated, may altogether reverse the effects of a potent drug. In studies with Methantheline Bromide, U.S.P. (Banthine, ß-diethylaminoethyl-9-xanthene-carboxylate methobromide), for example, it was determined that 100 mg of the agent powerfully inhibited gastric secretion with the maximum effect occurring approximately ninety minutes after oral ingestion. In repeated experiments after inhibition of gastric acid secretion by the agent had been achieved but before the maximum effect had occurred, an interview covering significant personal conflicts was undertaken. There was observed a brisk increase in gastric acid secretion above control levels despite the inhibitory effect of the methantheline bromide.

Cleghorn et al. (1950) were able significantly to activate adrenocortical activity with hypodermic injection of sterile saline. Rinzler et al. (1953) were able to effect a statistically significant reduction in the concentration of serum lipoproteins by the administration of placebos. All of these findings indicate simply that the responsible mechanisms are connected with circuits in the cerebral cortex.

The Placebo in Therapeutic Research

There is not universal agreement as to the place of the placebo in therapeutic research. Some investigators have asserted that the placebo control is unnecessary or even misleading (Batterman, 1955; Schroeder, 1955), but most agree that it is an indispensable step toward the establishment of the therapeutic efficacy of any new agent. The placebo by no means provides a perfect control procedure, however (Clauser, 1956; Clauser, 1957; Martini, 1957; Modell & Houde, 1949; Schelenz, 1958; Tuteur, 1958). Telltale side effects of a potent agent may vitiate the attempt to keep the physician or the subject unaware of what is being given. While placebos may induce almost any side effect, they do not produce them as predictably as does an active agent. Furthermore, the use of a placebo control may be awkward and cumbersome when establishing a dose range or when looking for serious toxic effects of an agent. In a clinical trial, however, and before the presumed therapeutic action of the agent can be accepted, the placebo must be given and given without the knowledge of either the one who gives it or the one who gets it because, as already pointed out, drug therapy backed by unconscious enthusiasm and solicitude of the physician may provide powerful and measurable bodily changes which are not attributable to the pharmacodynamic effects of the agent in question (Wolf, 1957). A case in point was that of a patient who had chronic asthma for twenty-seven years. Having suffered almost continuous asthma for the past seventeen, he had become a favorite subject on which to test new drugs. He had become refractory even to epinephrine. Finally, the product of one pharmaceutical company seemed effective in his case. When he was given the agent, he was free of asthma; when it was stopped, the asthma returned. Accordingly, his physician substituted a placebo without the patient's knowledge. Asthma was not relieved. Shifts from agent to placebo and back again were carried out several times with consistent results in favor of the agent. When the company was approached for an additional supply of the material, their representative acknowledged that, because they had had so much trouble with positive enthusiastic reports, they had, in this instance, sent along the placebo first. It would be hard to find a more vivid illustration of the need for placebo control to be blindly undertaken so that the doctor, as well as the patient, is ignorant of what is being administered. Investigators have often been naive in failing to recognize that patients, like dogs and children, are likely to know what is in the atmosphere without our telling them and even when we try desperately to conceal our attitudes.

Early enthusiastic reports of new pharmacodynamic agents rarely included placebo controls. Data on "tranquilizers" have provided no exception. From 1949 to 1953, numerous publications described the powers of mephenesin to reduce the subjective and objective manifestations of anxiety and tension. When these powers were tested with adequate controls, it was discovered that they did not exceed those of a placebo (Wolf & Pinsky, 1954).

In the evaluation of a new pharmacodynamic agent, the most relevant question is, "What is the agent being asked to accomplish?" Until recently, despite a great deal of literature on the "tranquilizers" and a good deal of earnest effort by honest investigators, we had only impressions and enthusiasms. It is well to remember that the man who first stumbled onto sulfur water in the first spa was also greatly impressed and enthusiastic about its curative properties. The sulfur water, so it seemed, proved highly efficacious for him and for others for many years. For many years people were relieved of various forms of arthritis, asthma, and other disorders when they drank these sulfurous waters or immersed themselves in them. People still go to spas, still improve vastly, but attribute the therapeutic effect to the restful atmosphere and don't bother with drinking or bathing in the water!

In every branch of therapeutics, including drug therapy and psychotherapy, we must take into consideration the accidental introduction of the really important therapeutic principle and of wrongly attributing the good result to an irrelevant factor. As DuBois wrote, "Any young neophyte can introduce a new drug. It requires a man of large experience and considerable reputation to destroy an old one" (DuBois, 1939).

It is important to emphasize, as pointed out by Lasagna that the use of a placebo control alone does not eliminate the bias of either the patient or physician in interpreting results. Neither will data from a placebo group substitute for the untreated control (Lasagna, 1955). According to Modell and Houde (1958):

> No simple device such as the double-blind technique will correct astigmatism or myopia in the examination of drugs. The blind will not lead the blind to a valid conclusion unless the method somehow also provides vision. It is our contention

that the evaluation of the effects of drugs in man is by no means simpler, nor does it permit a less rigorous method of examination, than the formal experiment with the laboratory animal. The methodology has a strict discipline of its own. A great danger in interpreting clinical evaluations lies in failure to recognize the meaninglessness of the negative answer when the method is not sufficiently sensitive for the purpose. The failure to demonstrate statistically significant differences between drugs or treatments is frequently misinterpreted to mean that no real differences exist.... However, when the differences are statistically insignificant, a high probability of their being due to chance does not rule out the possibility that they may be real or even important. Such an occurrence could simply result from an inadequate trial or from an insensitive method of evaluation which statistical analysis may not indicate.

Early during the antibiotic era, Haight applied a proper placebo control to his studies in the antibiotic field (Haight, 1952, 1954). He found that when sore throats and flu-like syndromes were unaccompanied by the presence of beta hemolytic streptococci in the throat, the course of the illness was no shorter in those patients treated with penicillin or erythromycin than those treated with placebo. Grossman and Masserman found in studying the analgesic and antirheumatic effects of aspirin, phenacetin and other agents, using a blind placebo technique that the placebo was usually just as effective as the agent. They also observed nearly the same percentage of untoward reactions from the placebos as from the agents (Masserman, 1954).

In view of all this, the need for double blind control seems essential in order to protect us from the welter of favorable reports in the literature of agents that are forgotten in a few years. But placebo control is equally essential in evaluating adverse reactions attributed to a drug. In studies of antihypertensive drugs given by mouth to ambulatory patients, Schapiro and Grollman found that one of their most troublesome and persistent "apresoline" headaches occurred in an individual who was getting placebo at the time (Shapiro & Grollman, 1953).

Placebo Effect of Surgery

Like the giving of drugs or the laying on of hands, surgery is often productive of powerful placebo effects. In the 1920s, the leading surgeons of the nation were congratulating themselves for having found a "procedure...sound in its principles, doing away as it does with fundamental factor (the pylorus) in the persistence of ulcer, permitting of the discharge of gastric contents into the duodenum where they belong and allowing alkaline duodenal contents to pass back into the stomach for neutralization of gastric acids" (Lahey, 1930). These words of Frank Lahey were spoken in the heat of the battle between the surgeons who advocated gastroenterostomy and those who recommended gastric resection for duodenal ulcer. At a symposium of the American Surgical Society, John Douglas reported 80 percent five-year cures in sixty-eight patients with duodenal ulcer who had been treated with gastroenterostomy for duodenal ulcer, a treatment that would be considered malpractice today. The powerful placebo effect of the operation is inherent in the fact Douglas found only 1.6 percent marginal ulcers among his patients while A.A. Berg, a surgeon who did not believe the value of the operation, was reporting a 33.33 percent incidence of marginal ulcer (Berg, 1930). Among powerful placebo personalities who had done well in treating duodenal ulcer by gastroenterostomy were Crile and Lord Moynihan and W.J. Mayo. The same sequence of innovation, early efficacy, enthusiasm, and then failure and disappointment, was experienced with such surgical procedures as thorcolumbarsympathectomy in the treatment of hypertension.

Detection of the Placebo Reactor

The measurable effects that may follow exhibition of a given agent, but are not attributable to its pharmacodynamic properties, at one time aroused the hope that those human subjects who frequently display placebo responses may be avoided by the investigator. Lasagna et al. (1954) described the placebo reactor as "a recognizable type, but only in the sense that intensive interview and psychologic testing can differentiate him from a nonreactor." Jellinek, in testing the effects of placebos and analgesics on headache, found that placebo reactors could be separated from non-reactors on a U-shaped curve (Jellinek, 1946). Other workers, on the other hand, were unable to adduce evidence that a placebo reactor was sufficiently characteristic to be identifiable even after six trials in an experimental situation (Wolf et al., 1957). Twenty-seven healthy young subjects were given ipecac, each on two occasions. The incidence of nausea among these individuals was 100 percent on both occasions. Most of them vomited both times. On seven successive occasions, however, after a premedication with a placebo, the situation changed. Nausea failed to occur in many instances. Many who did become nauseated felt that it was not so severe as it had been on the two original occasions. During the seven trials with placebo premedication, it was found that all of the subjects at one time failed to become nauseated and thereby showed a placebo reaction although it was not possible to predict, after several experiences, whether or not an individual would be more or less likely to show the placebo reaction. In fact, the pattern of distribution of placebo responses was identical with a chance distribution achieved by designating coins as subjects and flipping each coin seven times. Heads was called placebo response and tails, no response. The findings of the experiment were almost identical with those observed in the coin tossing (Wolf et al., 1957). In this study, the lack of predictability of the placebo reaction was evident. Furthermore, there was observed a lack of consistency in the way in which the various individuals responded to placebos.

The differences in the conclusions implied from the studies of the various workers may be reconciled in view of the evidence that placebo reactions depend upon the particular circumstances prevailing at each administration. Relevant among these would be the nature of the symptom being treated, the motivation of patient and physician, the nature of the test agent, its mode of administration and the life situation of the subject at the time he is tested. The significant point here is not the apparently conflicting findings of investigators with respect to placebo reactors, but rather that in any given situation, responses to a placebo may vary as compared to any other situation, and the significance of situations to human subjects cannot be precisely duplicated. Therefore, it seems unlikely that a placebo reactor can be identified and eliminated from an experimental situation on the basis of evidence gathered from some other situation. Rigorous placebo control will probably continue to be necessary in therapeutic research. Any new therapeutic maneuver may induce the desired effects in some subjects and may even be documented by quantitative viable changes in organ function.

The Place of the Placebo in Therapy

Placebo effects are probably the most relied upon aspects of pharmacotherapy today, however unintentional this may be on the part of the physician. The daily flood of samples and advertisements for nostrums that flows over the desk of every medical practitioner in the United States is proof enough. When the enthusiasm of the salesman is conveyed to the patients the need for rigorous testing is all the more evidence. Thus, in a sense, the question of whether or not to prescribe placebos is an academic one. As Modell has stated it (Modell, 1955), "No physician can correctly make a blanket statement that he never applies a placebo; he merely uses it involuntarily without knowledge or understanding. The question is not whether the physician should or should not use placebo, but how he should best utilize the always potentially present effect."

Gliedman et al. (1957) reported two groups of patients with bleeding ulcers treated with placebos. One group was told by the doctor that a new medicine would be given them which would undoubtedly produce relief. The other group was told by nurses that an experimental medicine would be administered, the effects of which were more or less unknown. In both instances, the same agent was employed, namely, the placebo. In the first group 70 percent of the patients had excellent results, while, in the second group, only 25 percent showed a favorable response.

Some authors have argued warmly in favor of the deliberate giving of placebos while others, fearing a diminution in emphasis on understanding of the patient as a person, have vigorously decried their use. The most frequently proposed indications are (1) in substitution for narcotic agents to allay anxiety and minimize the possibilities of addiction; (2) to administer to those who demand medication to tide them over until an effective relationship can be made for psychotherapy; (3) to test the effectiveness of therapeutic agents.

Placebo therapy should not be relied on too heavily. Although results are, at times, brilliant, they can hardly be expected to be either consistent or persistent. Perhaps the most satisfactory position on placebo therapy was taken by Perry Pepper (1945) who wrote, "The giving of a placebo—when, how, and what—seems to be a function of the physician which, like certain of the functions of the body, is not to be mentioned in polite society."[3]

Formulation

Nearly forty years ago G.W. Pickering referred to the controlled therapeutic trial as the most important medical development of the past ten years (Pickering, 1958). Recognition of the power and the properties of the placebo has been an important part of this development. Thus the placebo has gained a useful and more dignified place in the therapeutic armamentarium. As an inert placebo or a placebo in the form of a drug may ameliorate bodily disorders, so also may a host of rituals and procedures including surgery and a variety of forms of psychotherapy and so may the healing presence of the physician. It is important to realize that every contact with a physician is a meaningful situation to the patient, and, as such, may set off visceral responses that can have salutary or adverse effects on his health and well-being. To establish the intrinsic worth of any therapeutic agent or maneuver, a well-designed and properly controlled test situation is required. A proper therapeutic experiment requires skill, experience and sophistication.

Notes

1. The carefully designed protocol for the testing of antituberculosis drugs, sponsored and supervised by the Veterans Administration, became a model of research design. The findings, subjected as they were to painstaking analysis, provided for the first time, reliable efficacious treatments for tuberculosis in its various forms.
2. Tom, with his readily accessible stomach was studied for seventeen years before his death in 1958 (Wolf & Wolff, 1947; Wolf, 1965). A placebo, introduced into Tom's stomach when he thought he was being given a gastric stimulator, sharply increased gastric acid secretion and motor activity.
3. O.H. Perry Pepper, professor of medicine at the University of Pennsylvania and president of the College of Physicians of Philadelphia, found to his surprise, that his paper on the placebo was the first published according to the Index of the Surgeon General's Library (later to be known as the National Library of Medicine). He also noted that the word, *placebos*, had been used as the name of Vespers in the Office for the Dead in the Christian ritual science of the thirteenth century (Pepper, 1945).

9

Biological Integration and Synthesis

The foregoing chapters have identified some of the many physical and chemical structures and strategies that participate in the human biological adaptations that determine health or disease. They perform in interactive, dynamic systems of increasing levels of complexity. The most fundamental level of integration is concerned with survival and growth of tissue cells and communication among them. The next level is populated by circulating chemical agents that communicate among cells at a distance and thereby evoke specific thermodynamic behaviors such as oxidative phosphorylation, bone building and repair, and metabolism of nutrients. At a higher level of integration are the interactions of various regulatory minisystems including cellular (cytokines), glandular, (hormones, enzymes, ligands, and their receptors), and partially independent neuronal plexuses such as those that direct simple adaptive functions in the heart and gut.[1]

Elegant adaptive functions may be made independently at each of the above levels of integration. Even when isolated from the organism and placed in a suitable medium, cells and organs will carry out their functions for a time under the strict and immutable laws of thermodynamics and redox equilibrium.

The highest level of integration in man is the central nervous system that directly or indirectly controls not only the circulatory, gastrointestinal, endocrine, and immune functions, but also the distribution of receptors and ligands, the production of tropic and trophic substances in and around all the structures of the body, including the liver, kidney, spleen, bone marrow, reproductive organs and so on, allowing each of them to adjust to myriad internal and external challenges and changes. At the level of the whole organism, these structures are brought together in a collaborative adaptive and nonlinear neural hormonal and immunological regulatory process that, under the ultimate control of the brain, is capable of responding to perturbations of all sorts while maintaining life. Driving the entire complex of integrated systems are afferent signals from within and without the organism including adaptive demands from life experiences.

Discovering the Functions of the Brain

Despite a persisting general awareness of the role of the brain in initiating and patterning bodily reactions of all sorts, experimental access to the machinery of the brain seemed for centuries, unattainable. As late as the last century the distinguished Swedish scientist, Berzelius, in an 1813 publication, declared that no progress was possible in understanding the brain (Berzelius, 1813). Over a half a century later, Joseph Hyrtl, the great anatomist of Vienna predicted "The anatomy inside the brain is, and will probably always remain, a book closed with seven seals and written in hieroglyphics in addition" (Hyrtl, 1846). They, of course, had not allowed for the extraordinary technical advances that were to occur subsequently.

The brain mechanisms involved in regulating the bodily economy have been probed through measurements of behavior and various electroencephalographic, radiographic, and other experimental techniques, but knowledge of the mechanisms whereby the brain stores information and evaluates experience continues to be fragmentary. Early evidence of the storage of experiences in the brain came from the work of Wilder Penfield who, in his patients with temporal lobe epilepsy, found that sights, sounds, and happenings in the long past of their lives could, by appropriately applied electrical stimulation to the brain, be vividly reexperienced (Penfield, 1950). Current technical refinements have made it possible to explore, stimulate, and record from fairly precisely identified structures in the brain. From such studies it has become evident that, while the basic neuronal structures and their distribution in the brain is species specific, and to some extent specific to the individual, their fine dendritic development is epigenetic and is largely determined by experience (Buell & Coleman, 1979).

Neuronal Plasticity

Scheibel and colleagues made postmortem analyses of pyramidal neurons in various cortical receptive zones in the brains of individuals with differing levels of education and types of occupation. They revealed that the richness and patterns of dendritic development corresponded roughly to the cortical localization of the body parts most involved in their daily activities (Scheibel & Wechsler, 1990). Scheibel recalled observations of Oscar and Cecile Vogt made in 1954 (Scheibel & Wechsler, 1990). In autopsy specimens they had observed unusual thickness of the primary auditory receptive cortex of a violinist who in life had had perfect pitch. They had also observed enhancement of the primary visual cortex in an artist with extraordinary eidetic powers and comparable developments in the cortices of other highly talented individuals. Although such findings do not distinguish between genetic and developmental changes, Hubel and Wiesel have shown that visual experience is essential to the development of the visual cortex and furthermore that such sensory exposure must occur during a critical time period in infancy (Hubel & Wiesel, 1959, 1963). Although the techniques of measuring and tracing dendritic branching need a great deal more development, refinement, and precision before their physiological consequences and explanatory power can be stated, they nevertheless offer a hopeful step toward understanding the role of dendritic interactions in cognitive, emotional, and behavioral development.

Scheibel emphasized that inferences from such observations must be made from well-studied individuals rather than from combined data on groups: "Brain tissue is so sensitive a reflector of the inheritance, moods, activities, skills, and challenges of the individual that it is almost impossible to have too fine-grained a history of the subject if satisfactory correlations are to be attempted. In a sense, the neurostructural and neurochemical milieu are at once the cause and effect of the history of the individual...an organic autobiography" (Scheibel & Wechsler, 1990).

Developments thus far in the effort to identify the central neural structures involved in the evaluation of experience have shown that new sensory signals entering the appropriate receptive area (i.e., cochlear or solitary nucleus, thalamus, olfactory or optic cortex, etc.) activate a vast array of excitatory and inhibitory intracranial neurons that communicate and interact with several other sites in the brain, including the reticular activating system, locus ceruleus, hippocampus and identified areas of the insular, temporal, occipital, and frontal cortices. From vast numbers of neuronal interactions is recruited stored information consisting of beliefs, biases, aspirations, vulnerabilities, and essentially all that has been learned. Thus, with astounding speed, is achieved a strictly individual interpretation of the original sensory message (Brown, 1988; Deacon, 1988; Pandya & Yeterian, 1985; Scheibel & Wechsler, 1990). One such afferent system that interprets olfactory stimuli has been fairly well identified in rabbits by Gray, Freeman and Skinner 1986; (Skinner, 1990). Several other cortical connections of somatic and visceral sensory systems involving cardiovascular and other structures also have been partially traced (Mountcastle et al., 1984).

The Guiding Force of Experience

The more or less abstract message that is generated by the almost simultaneous interactions of millions of neurons directs an effector cascade that may involve activity in somatic, autonomic, immunologic, and endocrine effector mechanisms to produce discrete, patterned and purposeful visceral and somatic behaviors (Danielopolu, 1944; Wolf, 1970; Ornstein, 1990). These are consequences of experience that depend largely on the meaning of the event to the affected individual. The meaning to the individual therefore becomes the appropriate subject for study.

While modern biologists turn a blind eye to intangible evidence, the philosophers, who were the first to engage in formal inquiries into psychology, had no difficulty accepting meaning and significance as legitimate matters for study as readily as they did objective, observable phenomena. In the early eighteenth century, the famous philosopher and mathematician, Christian von Wolff proposed the existence of an intangible physical force at work in human interactions (Blackwell, 1961). Wolff had approached psychology with the concepts and methods of physics. He suggested that, as the explanation of physical phenomena is to be found in the laws of motion, so the interhuman force, capable of producing a somatic or visceral change, is reflective of individual experience, and especially of human interactions. As Claude Bernard put it: "The vital force directs phenomena that it does not produce; the physical agents produce phenomena they do not direct" (Bernard, 1839). As he used the term, vital, to distinguish living organisms from inanimate bodies, he was pointing out that the organism operates at all levels in response to its experience. It is the experience, then, that initiates the force that Bernard refers to, that is, a force that does not lend itself to the reductionistic analysis. Although irreducible, it is nevertheless comprehensible as a powerful and universal intangible. Thus, as significant as are the brain's intricate, versatile and elegant tangible structures and their awesome capacity to intercommunicate, it is specifically *how* the structures interrelate that determines the character of their product. As Hughlings Jackson put it: "Neural organization is dependent on, but distinct from anatomical structure" (Jackson, 1889).

Strategies of Inquiry

Since, depending on initial conditions, the influences of life experience may vary widely from person to person, the focus of inquiry must be on the individual person. While the structures and mechanisms capable of responding to experience are more or less uniform from person to person, the responses that they activate are epigenetic, influenced by development and experience and therefore potentially dissimilar. For example, faced with a threat to self-esteem, one individual may, because of past life experiences unique to him or her, respond with a sharp rise in blood pressure, an outpouring of acid gastric juice or other physiologic disturbances while another individual, responding to the same circumstance, may experience a fall in blood pressure and collapse in a faint or experience nausea associated with inhibition of gastric motility and secretion (Wolf, 1980, 1985). Negoescu and colleagues, in a study of the contrasting effects of intellectual effort and relaxation on the amplitude of sinus arrhythmia found that the outcome in either state could be predicted only with knowledge of each individual's preoccupations at the time (Negoescu et al., 1987).

The key to characterizing an individual is to ascertain his or her weltanschauung, one's way of looking at life. Such information may be available in a skillfully conducted dialogue but is less accessible from uniform predesigned paper and pencil tests, which cannot detect subtleties that distinguish us from one another. Neither can contrived presumably stressful stimuli be expected to impose a standardized impact on an experimental subject.[2] Mental arithmetic, a relatively stable favorite, though onerous or even frightening to some, is fun for others. Further progress will require new questions framed to conform to the determinative nature of experience, the central processing of which produces individual, subjective interpretations that shape behavior. The potentially powerful force of words, gestures, music, art, or an idea on a person must, to be effective, encounter a receptor. Just as a tree falling in the forest makes noise only if the air waves it creates encounter a suitable detector, so the force that Wolff suggested has reality only if it engages the evaluative neuronal circuitry in the brain of one or more other human beings. Thus, the effect depends entirely on how the event is processed in the neural circuitry peculiar to the recipient or recipients.

Learning and Behavior

The ability to alter behavior to protect against a hostile environment can be found in some plants and trees that, once attacked by a predator, can protect themselves against subsequent attack by altering to some extent their tissue chemistry. Even single-celled organisms, paramecia, for instance, can learn to avoid previous sources of harm in stereotypic ways that do not involve many alternatives or choices. So also can lower invertebrates with simple neural networks. The learned behavior of invertebrates with more complex neural circuits, however, may vary with contingencies, as illustrated by the studies of electrophysiological interactions of identified neurons in aplysia and other mollusks. Their complex reflex functions require an organized neuronal circuit with the capacity to select a response among alternatives, as beautifully demonstrated by Kandel and his collaborators (Kandel, 1976; Pinsker, 1970). Bailey and Chen showed that morphologic changes accompany long-term habituation and sensitization in aplysia (Bailey & Chen, 1983). Such changes appear to be fundamental to neural plasticity that underlies the ability to select a behavior appropriate to the impact of specific circumstances. Nevertheless, the learned responses of aplysia are still stereotyped in the sense that they are monotonously predictable and uniform from organism to organism. Only in higher vertebrates, dogs, for instance, may a behavioral adaptation to an identical set of circumstances vary from animal to animal and even from time to time in the same animal. Thus, a "choice" of behavior becomes available thanks to the complex processing of experience in the highly ramified mammalian nervous system. In humans we see the emergence of judgment and discrimination as well as language, beliefs, and intellectual interests.

Pinsker and Willis in 1980 published the proceedings of an interdisciplinary conference that attempted a synthesis of separate and sometimes disparate findings of neurobiologists, psychologists, mathematician-engineers, clinicians, and philosophers concerning the workings of the nervous system and its implications for understanding human behavior (Pinsker & Willis, 1980). This rich resource provides links between levels of neural organization from molecular to behavioral. The book deals with the increased complexity of organization that allows an organism to perform more abstract and less precisely definable functions, characteristics of individual human personalities and to endow the individual with qualities such as courage, honesty, loyalty, generosity, and creative imagination.

Intangible Forces and Functions

An intriguing view of the functions of the brain beyond maintaining life, health, and vigor, is found in the writings of Paracelsus (Theophrastus Bombastus Von Hohenheim) an early sixteenth-century physician and natural philosopher who considered the brain to be an expressive instrument or device, not a cause of intellectual or emotional behavior. From his *De Veribus Morborum*, his biographer, Hartman quotes: "Wisdom, reason and thought are not contained in the brain, but thus belong to the invisible universal spirit which feels through the heart and thinks by means of the brain. All these powers...become manifest through material organs" (Paracelsus, 1891).

Paracelsus seemed to be suggesting that the brain, like a violin, trumpet, flute, or guitar, is an instrument, albeit a living instrument, that is capable of giving rise to thoughts, emotions, aspirations, and behavior. As the nature and quality of music depends in part on the characteristics of the instrument, so the nature and quality of the products of a brain depend on its characteristics and the afferent data fed into it. Recent studies of senile dementia of the Alzheimer type have reawakened an old concern with the significance of sensory input to the maintenance of intellectual functioning. The idea that sensory information contributes in a major way to shaping the structure of the brain and is a fundamental requirement for mental activity took root in the seventeenth century with Pierre Gassendi and John Locke. Later in France Pierre Jean George Cabanis, professor of medicine in the Faculté de Medecine in Paris, began to evolve a unified concept of the mind-body relationship based on physiology (Cabanis, 1981). He propounded the idea that not only thoughts and emotions, but also general, somatic, and visceral behavior are individually shaped by life experiences perceived through the senses and influenced by stored information from earlier experiences as well as by the structure and capability of each individual brain.

Intelligence

Cabanis was also aware that the organization of the brain, established through genetic inheritance, epigenetic development, and life experience, endows individuals with differing capacities and talents, thereby making possible a rich variety of human achievement which, in turn, requires the influence of intangibles such as interest, aspirations, determination, esthetic sense, curiosity, and so on. Intangible music, produced by tangible musical instruments, may exert effects powerful enough to influence the behavior of people and even the course of events in history. [3] So may the intangible thoughts of man when spoken or written and preserved for posterity. The pen, being more powerful than the sword, may maintain its influence indefinitely.

Notes

1. The Auerbach and Meissner plexuses located respectively in the intestinal muscle and submucosa are, by virtue of their local circuits containing afferent neurons, interneurons, and efferent neurons, capable of regulating some functions of the gut independent of the central neural connections. The heart's intrinsic regulatory plexus is identifiable in the fat pads located on its surface. The interactive neurons that comprise this intrinsic regulator extend throughout the myocardium. Some of the basic studies on this system have been done by Andrew Armour and his colleagues (Armour, 1993).
2. Differences in perception of a stimulus from person to person and even from time to time in the same subject have been widely documented. Nevertheless, "standardized" stress stimuli continue to be relied on in much psychological research. The physiological and behavioral responses to a stimulus are far more replicable in animals than in humans.
3. The effect of the "Marseillaise" during the French Revolution is a powerful example of the social influence of music. "Giovinezza" during the rule of Mussolini in Italy is another and the "strength through joy" youth songs in Nazi Germany under Hitler is a third. At a more civilized level, "We Shall Overcome" was a powerful spur to the antisegregation movement in the United States.

Afterword

The objective of this book has been to examine in historical perspective, the current state of medical education, research, and practice and to encourage the medical establishment to focus more sharply on the needs of the patient as opposed to a general conception of "health care." Scanning the past millenium reveals cycles of major changes in how to educate physicians. For example, the practice of teaching students at the bedside has either had a high priority or, from time to time, has been ignored. Giovanni Battista Da Monte (1498–1551) introduced bedside teaching of students at the hospital of San Francisco in Padua. After his death the practice died out in Italy, was revived in Leiden, in the Netherlands, enjoyed popularity in Edinburgh, Paris, and then successively in Canada, The United States, and England under William Osler (Altschule, 1989). Today bedside teaching is suffering neglect.[1] The philosophical approach to medical education has vacillated widely since Hippocrates, during the golden age of Greece, wrote: "Medicine is the most distinguished of all arts" (Hippocrates, *Law* Bk. I). He also extolled the importance of science as the road to knowledge (Hippocrates, Bk. IV). His work had been preceded by the natural history studies of Aristotle in the fourth century B.C.

After the writings of Hippocrates the next real text on medicine was produced by Aulus Cornelius Celsus, backed by the Roman Emperor, Tiberius, in about 30 A.D. Thereafter there appeared several treatises on *materia medica* in Italy, Greece, and Egypt.[2]

Until the early 1900s, medical practice in America was essentially a loosely regulated craft. Thereafter, following the publication of the Flexner report in 1912,[3] American medicine enjoyed a period of scholarly development and rapid progress toward world leadership. Medical education had emerged from an informal apprenticeship to a highly organized process of schooling and hospital training with close relationships between professor and student. For several years medical research continued to be based on the study of sick patients until recently when patients became the subject of surveys and epidemiological inquiries, largely replacing patient-oriented laboratory research. Current laboratory investigations are carried out mainly at the level of genes, molecules, and cells with the confident hope that a reductionistic approach will yield understanding of the biological dynamics that underlie states of health and disease. As rich as has been the yield from molecular biology and genetics, the study and care of the sick still require a combination of art and science at a more highly integrated level of inquiry.

Since World War II both medical research and practice have attracted public interest of increasing intensity. Education, research, and practice have become more highly organized, thus contributing to the process of making our society more bureaucratic, more managed and less flexible. As "management" has been presumed to be the problem solver, medical faculties have become occupied with visits from accrediting bodies to medical schools and their hospitals and with planning and curriculum committees being overseen by a constantly enlarging corps of administrators. As a consequence, there is less time in the day for potentially inspirational personal contacts between faculty leaders and young, aspiring doctors. The medical school experience has consequently become less fulfilling, less fun.

The government-mandated enlargement of the student body has also contributed to the increasingly impersonal atmosphere of the medical schools. The traditional, highly valuable "out of hours" learning in the laboratories, on the wards, and in the emergency room has been seriously curtailed by another social shift. Prior to World War II, few medical students, interns, or residents were married. Some university hospitals would not accept married interns and required interns and residents to live in the hospital building where countless opportunities for learning were at hand. After the war, for the first time, a large percentage of the medical students were married with family responsibilities and demands. Since interns and residents were no longer housed in the hospital, it became necessary for teaching hospitals to provide them a living wage. Persistently, financial problems intruded to the disadvantage of the educational process. The flood of new diagnostic and therapeutic technology, valuable as they were, required a progressive increase in technical and nursing personnel, more space and more time. The size of medical school administration and faculties increased rapidly and at considerable cost. NIH grants for research that initially prohibited support for faculty salaries began to support full salaries for those involved with research and eventually went on to cover "indirect" costs for the host institution in amounts varying up to 100 percent of the cost of the research itself. Many of the faculty members became sequestered in laboratories, thus having very little contact with students. Ultimately, financial pressures on medical schools caused the "full time" teaching faculty to engage in private practice in competition with physicians in their community, a further impairment of potentially inspirational contacts between students and their professors.

The practice of medicine also fell victim to financial exigencies owing in part to escalating costs of insurance policies, of managing the paperwork required by third-party payers, and the cost of the profits due to those agencies. Beyond that was the cost of compensating the doctors, the private agencies, and the regulatory government agencies for the provision of medical care to the disadvantaged. Such economic difficulties have encouraged the ultimate commercialization of medicine. Large for-profit corporations are already acquiring and operating university medical centers and community hospitals as well. To maintain a flow of patients and profits to the hospitals the proprietor companies have been purchasing the practices of previously independent physicians in the region and have put them on salary with requirements to treat an established minimum of patients or perform a minimum of surgical operations.

Extracting a viable and helpful system from this social, financial, and political morass in which the provision of medical care to the people finds itself will require a careful re-reexamination of medicine's mission, the needs of medical education, research, and practice and thoughtful consideration of strategies to achieve them. While the financial imperative must be dealt with, it should not crowd out the mission as the central goal.

The Mission

The main responsibility of medical schools is to graduate students who, with a generous spirit and a high degree of competence, are dedicated primarily to understanding and caring for their patients. The first step toward achieving this goal is the selection of candidates for medical school who are of good character as well as being intellectually and emotionally qualified. During the school years the goal must be to stimulate learning and to inspire the students toward an appetite for inquiry and dedication to service in order to meet the needs of the public. The schools are presently producing a 2 to 1 majority of high-tech specialists over general internists and pediatricians. The imbalance may be due to the already mentioned reduced opportunities for individual relationships with faculty members who, with a broad command of medicine, exemplify the intellectual, emotional, and spiritual rewards of the "thinking doctor." This type of physician, embodied by William Osler, and once known as a diagnostician, is a rare species today that needs to be revived.

This daunting challenge calls for the wisdom to achieve adequate and appropriate financial support for medical education, while still maintaining a primary focus on the individual, on education, medical research, and on the care of patients. This wisdom will not be extracted from the reflections of political planners, of scientists focused on a single line of inquiry, of closeted administrators, or of advocates in medical organizations. These and other groups must be heard, but the recommendations must come from seasoned observers who have seen and felt the force of the trends and policies that have affected young aspirants to a medical career, their teachers, their schools and hospitals and have dealt with the problems related to the selection of research projects for financial support.

The present arrangements in all three spheres are far from ideal, are not even satisfactory. It is likely that the needed revolution will emerge from the thinking of a single person or from a small group of persons, as did the very different kind of medical revolution set off by Flexner. Such an urgently needed achievement will require the initiative of a few wise heads and the understanding and support of the people.

A few years ago in France, an organization was established under the leadership of Gaston Berger. It was called "Prospective." The group's deliberations, focused not on medicine, but on the whole spectrum of social development, were brought together in a publication called *Shaping the Future* (Cournand & Lévy, 1973). These Frenchmen held that, while one cannot predict the future, one should be able to do three things— to sense what "is coming down the pike" in terms of trends for the near future, to prepare for such predictable new developments and, to some extent, to influence their character, that is, to shape the future.[4]

Delivering Health Care? Or Caring for the Patient?

In current discussions of the future of medicine in the Congress, the press and even in publications of medical societies, medicine has become "health care," doctors are "health care providers." "The medical market place" describes medical practice. As Leon Eisenberg (1995) commented in a thoughtful editorial:

Medical care is being "monitorized"; physicians are becoming the "proletarians" of health care capitalism. The lexicon of our hospitals is rife with terms borrowed from the corporate world: teaching hospitals "position themselves" to seize their "market share," "demarket" money-losing clinical services, diversify, "unbundle," "spin-off" for-profit subsidiaries, develop "convenience-oriented feeder systems," maneuver to adjust case mix, and triage admissions by their ability to pay and "deselect" physicians with costly styles of practice.

An incisive analysis of such "managerial care" has recently been provided by Caroline Poplin, a practicing physician with a strong legal background (Poplin, 1995). The commercialization of medicine appears to stem in large part from the high cost of the multitude of technical innovations in diagnosis and therapy and perhaps in part from their over use. Overdependence on such measures by physicians has doubtless contributed to shortening the dialogue between physician and patient and to giving their encounter an impersonal quality. Modern medical technology has become not only a time saver, but a thought saver as well. The rapid development of dependence on technology was examined in a Totts Gap Colloquium. *The Technological Imperative in Medicine* in 1981 (Wolf & Berle, 1981).

One prediction made at the colloquium was that there would be a trend toward more group associations among physicians. During the succeeding years HMOs have multiplied and costs of medical care have escalated. Since neither physicians nor government have, in the spirit of "Prospective," evolved a plan for providing comprehensive medical care at affordable prices, perhaps a few remaining leading lights in medicine should sense the opportunity to be proactive instead of reactive and to participate in shaping the future. It is time for the thinkers to emerge, but none have done so. Instead, the acquisitive power of the commercial world has largely taken over.

The commercialization of medical practice and medical education has advanced to th epoint where, insurance, pharmaceutical companies, and other entrepreneurial organizations are merging and purchasing medical schools and their university hospitals. Community hospitals are buying the practices of local physicians, and requiring the doctors to make referrals only to their hospital staffs. The staff physicians and surgeons are required to adhere to limitation of diagnostic and therapeutic measures that are deemed "cost effective" by their owners and to treat a prescribed number of patients each day. Surgeons may lose staff privileges if they fail to perform at least a minimum number of certain procedures per year.

The consequences of this pattern of medical practice, called managed care, is to expose patients to the risk of cursory diagnostic and therapeutic attention, a restricted range of tests, medications, and other treatments dictated by cost-conscious medical administrators to insure a profit to the owner company. These and other restrictions go to extremes in some managed care arrangements, prohibiting reimbursement to a patient who has consulted a physician outside the group, even for a second opinion concerning a hazardous surgical procedure.

Perhaps the most dangerous impact of the system is on the quality of education of medical students. The senior full-time medical faculty who once spent their day with the students are now required to see private patients or are immersed in research laboratories. An attempt to meet the challenge in a small way is being made by Totts Gap Institute through a novel "role model" program aimed at developing broadly-oriented leaders in medicine. Totts Gap was founded in 1958 as a summer research laboratory. Until 1995 the institute's principal function was to provide young physicians an opportunity to engage in integrative physiological and clinical research.[5]

The strategy of the new program is to start cultivating leadership at a younger age, during the summer of the junior or senior year of high school. The program was begun in 1995 in collaboration with the Oklahoma School of Science and Mathematics. Six students, three young women and three young men who had opted for a career in medicine were selected by the faculty to spend seven weeks at Totts Gap. With a faculty of four widely experienced physician-scientists and two distinguished basic scientists, the students were introduced to the ethics of medical research and practice, to the necessary intellectual and personal qualities requisite to leadership in medicine. In tutorial sessions a member of the faculty worked with one or more students who reported on assigned reading, shared in the past experiences of the teacher and engaged in dialogue dealing with the broad intellectual, behavioral, and scientific issues related to medical research and to the understanding and care of the patient. Scattered among the formal sessions were less structured encounters between the students and teachers at the swimming pool, on the tennis court, on rafts in the Delaware River, during weekend outings to Philadelphia or New York museums or to observe ward rounds at nearby Universities.

Each of the students was asked to design a small experimental project to pursue independently under the oversight and encouragement of one of the faculty. Each project was completed, presented orally, and written by the student as a proper manuscript.

The whole undertaking was highly successful from the standpoint of the students, the Oklahoma School of Science and Mathematics, and Totts Gap. Whether or not such a program will contribute toward decomercialization and debureaucratizating medicine, at the same time encouraging scholarship, dedication, and selflessness within the profession we cannot predict.

Since the objective of our program was to influence young aspirants to a career in medicine, and since the beginning effort was small, we called the project "Brighten the Corner," hoping that close relationships between student and teacher, as a strategy toward learning and character development, would influence other institutions and ultimately resupply dedicated, broadly oriented role models and leaders to the medical faculties, the biological scientists, and practicing physicians of the nation.

Notes

1. Hoping to revive and perpetuate the Oslerian tradition in America, a group of outstanding physician-teachers formed the American Osler Society. It meets yearly in association with either the American College of Physicians or the American Society for the History of Medicine. The founders were: William Bean, Alfred Henderson, George Harrell, Thomas Durant, and Terry Cavanagh. The first honorary members were Wilbert Davidson and Wilder Penfield.
2. Aretaeus of Cappodocia and others wrote mainly descriptions of diseases in the early second century A.D. Then came the clinical and anatomical studies of Galen and later, in the seventh century, the surgical and medical studies of Paulus of Aegina. A major exponent of Greco-Arabic medicine was Avicenna (980–1037). Some of the first organized scientific research was done by a German aristocrat and polymath Christian bishop Albertus Magnus (1193–1280) of Cologne, the teacher of Thomas Aquinas who was later sainted. Research in medicine picked up momentum in the fifteenth and sixteenth centuries with a boost from Leonardo da Vinci. The long-standing anatomical dogmas of Galen finally became superannuated by the work of Jean Fernel (1497–1558) and Vesalius (1514–1564) and, by the late sixteenth and early seventeenth centuries, physiology was introduced by William Harvey (1578–1657). Soon thereafter modern chemistry began to dis-

place alchemy, thanks to the work of van Helmont (1614–1699), Thomas Willis (1621–1675) and Thomas Sydenham (1624–1689). These pioneers were soon joined by growing numbers of medical scientists throughout Europe.

The eighteenth century was blessed by substantial research achievements in rapid succession and, by the nineteenth, biomedical research had reached maturity. Contributions since then have grown exponentially. Recent advances, however, have depended more on technology than on extraordinary new insights. Thus, while the curve of progress has become progressively steeper, during the past thirty years it has become narrower, largely restricted by reductionistic thinking.

3. The American educator, Abraham Flexner, under the auspices of the Carnegie Foundation for the Advancement of Teaching, conducted an investigation of resources, programs, and curriculums of the medical schools throughout the U.S. The study, published in 1912, led to widespread reforms in many existing medical schools and the decease of others.

4. Gaston Berger, a French philosopher and sociologist, recognizing the futility of trying to predict the future, organized the Prospective Center in 1943 to develop and teach ways of sensing the direction of the future, devising strategies to adapt to it and possibly to modify the trend to some extent. André Cournand, a distinguished American physiologist and physician, joined the center in 1958 and edited their book with Maurice Lévy, *Shaping the Future* published in English in 1958. He also contributed a chapter on the application of prospective philosophy to medical education.

5. Totts Gap is an independent not-for-profit research institute located beneath the Appalachachian ridge in eastern Pennsylvania, equidistant, 65 miles north of Philadelphia and west of New York City. Originally a summer laboratory for research and training, it has operated year around since 1970.

Bibliography

Abbott, F.K., Mack, M., Wolf, S. "The relation of sustained contraction of the duodenum to nausea and vomiting." *Gastroenterology* 20 (1952):238–48.

Adams, W.F. *Ireland and Irish Emigration to the New World.* New Haven, CT: Yale University Press, 1932.

Ader, R., ed. *Psychoneuroimmunology.* New York: Academic Press, 1983.

Ahrens, E.H. *The Crisis in Clinical Research.* New York: Oxford University Press, 1992.

Akwa, Y., Morfin, R.F., Robel, P., Baulieu, E.E. "Neurosteroid metabolism. 7 alpha-hydroxylation of dehydroepiandrosterone and pregnenolone by rat microsomes." *Biochemistry Journal* 288 (1992):959–64.

Altschule, M. *Essays on the Rise and Decline of Bedside Medicine.* Philadelphia, PA: Lea & Febiger, 1989.

Andrews, C.H. "Propagation of Common Cold Virus in Tissue Cultures." *Lancet* 11 (1953):546.

Armour, J.A., Huang, M.H., Smith, F.M. "Peptidergic Modulation of In Situ Canine Intrinsic Cardiac Neurons." *Peptides* 14 (1993):191–202.

Association of American Medical Colleges book on Clinical Teaching. Physicians for the Twenty-First Century, Washington, DC, 1984

Astrow, A.B. "The French Revolution and the Dilemma of Medical Training." *Perspectives in Biology and Medicine* 33:3 (1990):444–45.

Bacon, P. *The New Organon and Related Writings.* New York: Liberal Arts Press, 1960.

Bailey, C.H., Chen, M. "Morphological Basis of Long-Term Habituation and Sensitization in Aplasia." *Science* 220 (1983):219–21.

Bard, P. and Woods, J.W. *The Physiologist*, vols. 2–3, August, 1959.

Barnes, R., Schottstaedt, W.W. "Abstract." *Clinical Research* 6 (1958):224.

Barr, D.P. "Hazards of modern diagnosis and therapy—the price we pay." *Journal American Medical Association* 159 (1955):1452–56.

Batterman, R.C. "Appraisal of new drugs." *Journal American Medical Association* 158 (1955):1547.

Bean, W.B. *Walter Reed: A Biography.* Charlottesville: University of Virginia, 1982.

Beaumont, W. *Experiments and Observations on the Gastric Juice and the Physiology of Digestion.* Plattsburg, NY: F.P. Allen, 1833.

Béclard, M.J. "Rapport général sur les prix décernés en 1862." *Academie de Médecine Paris* 26 (1863):xxxii–xiviii.

Bedell, S.E., Deitz, D.C., Leeman, D., Delbanco, T.L. "Incidence and characteristics of preventable iatrogenic cardiac arrests." *Journal American Medical Association*, 265 (1991):2815–20.

Beecher, H.K. "The powerful placebo." *Journal American Medical Association* 159 (1955):1602–06.

Beecher, H.K. "Evidence for increased effectiveness of placebos with increased stress." *American Journal of Physiology* 187 (1956):163–69.

Belkin, B.M., Neelon, F.A. *The Art of Observation: William Osler and the Method of Zadig*. In press.

Benet, S. *Abkhasians: The Long Living People of the Caucasus*. New York: Holt, Rinehart and Winston, 1965.

Berg, A.A. "The mortality and late results of subtotal gastrectomy for the radical cure of gastric and duodenal ulcer." *Annals of Surgery* 92 (1930): 340–59.

Berle, A.A. *The American/Economic Republic*. New York: Harcourt, Brace & World, 1963.

Bernard, C. *An Introduction to the Study of Experimental Medicine*. New York: Macmillan, 1926.

Bert, P. *Leçons sur la physiologie comparée de la respiration*. Paris: Baillière, 1879.

Berzelius, J.J. (1913). "A View of the Progress and Present State of Aromal Chemistry." In: Karczmer, A.G. Eccles, J.C. (eds.): *Brain and Human Behavior*, New York: Springer-Verlag, 1972.

Bett, W.R. *The History and Conquests of Communicable Diseases*. Norman: University of Oklahoma Press, 1954.

Bilisoly, E.N., Goodell, H., Wolff, H.G. "Vasodilation, lowered pain threshold, and increased tissue vulnerability. Effects dependent upon peripheral nerve function." *Archives of Internal Medicine* (Chicago) 94:759–73, 1954.

Black, P. McL. "Must Physicians Treat the "Whole Man" for Proper Medical Care?" *The Pharos*, January, 1976:8–11.

Blackwell, R.J. "Christian Wolff's doctrine of the soul." *Journal of the History of Ideas* 22 (1961):339–354.

Blattner, R.J., Heyes, F.M. "Pediatrics." In *Annual Review of Medicine*, Stanford, CA: Annual Reviews, Inc., 1956.

Bogdonoff, M.: "A brief look at medical grand rounds." *The Pharos* 45(1) (1982):16–18.

Boorstin, D.J. "Remarks by Daniel J. Boorstin, Librarian of Congress, at the White House Conference on Library and Informative Services." *Spec Libr* 71 (1980):113–16.

Brambelle, F., Racogni, G., De Wied, S. *Psychoneuroendocrinology: Proceedings of the XI Conference of International Society for Psychoneuroendocrinology.* New York: Elsevier-North Holland, 1980.

Brazier, M.A.B. (ed.). *The Central Nervous System and Behavior.* New York: Josiah Macy, Jr. Foundation, 1959.

Brown, J.W. *The Life of the Mind: Selected Papers.* Hilldale, NJ: Erlbaum, 1988.

Browning, R. "Andrea del Sarto." *Men and Women.* London: Chapman and Hall, 1855.

Bruhn, J.G., Wolf, S. "Studies reporting 'low rates' of ischemic heart disease. A critical review." *American Journal of Public Health* 8 (1970):1477–95.

Bruhn, J.G., Wolf, S. "Studies reporting "low rates" of ischemic heart disease: a critical review." *American Journal of Public Health* 60 (1970):1477–95.

Bruhn, J.G., Wolf, S. *The Roseto Story.* Norman: University of Oklahoma Press, 1979.

Brunner, D. Personal communication, 1968.

Buell, S.J., Coleman, P.D. "Dendritic growth in the aged human brain and failure of growth in senile dementia." *Science*, 206 (1979), 854–56.

Buller, A.J., Eccles, J.C., Eccles, R.M. *Journal of Physiology* 198 (1960): 669.

Burton, R. *Anatomy of Melancholy.* London: Chatto & Windus, 1891.

Bykov, K.M. *The Cerebral Cortex and the Internal Organs.* Trans. W. Horsely Gantt, New York: Chemical Publishing Co., 1957.

Cabanis, P.J.G. *On the Relations between the Physical and Moral Aspects of Man,* vol. 1, Saidi, M.D., trans., Mora, G., ed. Baltimore, MD: Johns Hopkins University Press, 1981.

Calvert, D.N., Brody, T.M. "Role of Sympathetic Nervous System in CCI_4 Hepatotoxicity." *American Journal of Physiology* 198 (1960):669.

Cannon, W.B. "Physiological regulation of normal states. Some tentative postulates concerning biological homeostatics." In *Richet, C. Ses Amis, Ses Collegues, Ses Elèves.* August Pettit, ed. Paris: Imprimerie des Editions Médicale. 1926, pp. 91–93.

Cannon, W.B. *Bodily Changes in Pain, Hunger, Fear, and Rage,* second edition. New York: Appleton, 1929.

Carvallo, J.L. "Estomac," In: Richet, C. *Dictionnaire de Physiologie,* vol. 5, 1902, pp. 849–54.

Cassel, E.G. *The Place of Humanities in Medicine.* Hastings on Hudson, NY: Hastings Center, 1984.

Castle, W.B. "Acceptance of the Kober Medal Award for 1962." *Transactions of the Association of American Physicians* 74 (1962):54–57.

Chamberlin, T.C. *Journal of Geology.* 1897, 5:837.

Chapman, L.F., Goodell, H., Wolff, H.G. "Augmentation of the inflammatory reaction by activity of the central nervous system." *Archives of Neurology* 1 (1959): 557-82.

Charon, R., Banks, J.T., Connelly, J.E., Hawkins, A.H., Hunter, K.M., Jones, A.H., Montello, M., Poirer, S. "Literature and Medicine: Contributions to Clinical Practice."
Annals of Internal Medicine 122 (1995):599–606.

Clauser, G. "Zur Kritik de sogenannten doppelten Blindversuchs in der Arzneimittelprüfung." *Med. Klinik* 51 (1956):1403–04.

Clauser, G. Klein, J. "Kritische Übersicht über das Plazeboproblem." *Münch. med. Wschr.* 99(1957):896–901.

Cleghorn, R.A., Graham, B.F., Campbell, R.P., Rublee, N.K., Elliot, F.H. Safran, M. "Anxiety states: Their response to ACTH and to isotonic saline." In: *Proceedings First Clinical ACTH Conference* Philadelphia, PA: Blakiston, 1950, pp. 561–555.

Clendening, L. *Source Book of Medical History*. Toronto: General Publishing Co., 1960.

Coburn, A.F. *Association of American Physicians* 73 (1960):669.

Cochran, W.G. "Research Techniques in the Study of Human Beings." *Milbank Memorial Fund Quarterly*, 33 (1955):121.

Cohnheim, J.F. *Lectures on General Pathology*. London: The New Syndeham Society, 1890.

Conn, J.W. "Some Clinical and Climatological Aspects of Aldosteronism in Man." *Transactions of the American Clinical and Climatological Association* 74 (1962).

Corvisart, N. In: *Source Book of Medical History,* edited by L. Clendening, Toronto: General Publishing Co., 1960, p. 306.

Cournand, A. (ed). *Shaping the Future*. New York, London, Paris: Gordon and Breach Science Publishers, 1973.

D'Angelo, S.A. *Journal of Endocrinology* 17 (1958):286.

Danielopolu, D. "Le Système Nerveux de la vie végétative." In: *Thérapeutique Médicale et Chirurgicale*. Paris: Masson, 1944.

Daniels, G.E. *Psychosomatic Medicine* I (1939):527.

Dantzler, W.H. "Regulatory Integrative and Comparative Physiology." *Perspectives American Journal of Physiology* 260 (1991):1021.

Darwin, C. *Origin of Species*. New York: P.F. Collier & Son, 1859.

Dawson, J. "Editorial." *Computers in Medicine* 11 (1982):1–3.

Daynes, R.A., Araneo, B.A., Ershler, W.B., Maloney, C., Li, G.Z., Ryu, S.Y. "Altered regulation of IL-6 production with normal aging. Possible linkage to the age-associated decline in dehydroepiandrosterone and its sulfated derivative." *Journal of Immunology* 150 (1993):5219–30.

Deacon, T. "Holism and Associationism in Neuropsychology. An Anatomical Synthesis." In: *Integrating Theory and Practice in Clinical Neurophysiology.* Hilldale, NJ: Erlbaum, 1988.

Denis, J.B. "A Letter Concerning a New Way of Curing Sundry Diseases by Transfusion of Blood." Written to M. de Montmor, London, 1667.

Dennis, L.B. *Psychology of Human Behavior for Nurses.* Philadelphia, PA: Saunders, 1957.

Descartes, R. *Discours de la Méthode pour Bien Conduire la Raison et Chercher la verité dans les Sciences.* Paris: Theodore Girard, 1668.

Dewhurst, K. *John Locke (1632–1704) Physician and Philosopher: A Medical Biography.* London: Wellcome Historical Medical Library, 1963.

Diehl, H.S. "Medicinal treatment of the common cold." *Journal American Medical Association* 101(1933):2042–49.

Diehl, H.S., Baker, A.B., Cowan, D.W. "Cold vaccines: A further evaluation." *Journal American Medical Association* 115 (1940):593–94.

Doig, R.K., Wolf, S., Wolff, H.G. "Study of gastric function in a "decorticate" man with gastric fistula." *Gastroenterology* 23 (1953):40–44.

Donnison, C.P. *Civilization and Disease.* Baltimore, MD: William Wood & Co, 1938.

Douglas, J. "Discussion of papers on mortality and late results of operations for gastric and duodenal ulcers." *Annals of Surgery* 92 (1930):631–34.

Drake, M.E. "Studies on Agent of Infectious Hepatitis." *Journal of Experimental Medicine* 95 (1952):231.

Drolet, G.J. "Epidemiology of Tuberculosis." In: *Clinical Tuberculosis.* B. Goldberg (ed.) Philadelphia, PA: F.A. Davis, 1946.

DuBois, E.F. "Elimination of worthless drugs." *Transactions Association of American Physicians* 54 (1937):1–5.

Dubos, R.J. "The Tubercle Bacillus and Tuberculosis." *American Scientist* 37 (1948):353.

Dubos, R.J. "Biological and Social Aspects of Tuberculosis." *Bulletin New York Academy of Medicine* 27 (1951):351.

Dubos, R.J., Dubos, J. *The White Plague: Tuberculosis, Man and Society.* Boston: Little, Brown and Co., 1952.

Dubos, R.J. *Mirage of Health.* New York: Harper & Brothers, 1959.

Duesberg, P.H. "AIDS epidemiology: Inconsistencies with human immunodeficiency virus and with infectious disease." *Proceedings National Academy of Science* 88 (1991):1575–79.

Dunbar, H.F. *Emotions and Bodily Changes,* second edition. New York: Columbia University Press, 1938.

Dunlop, C.W. *Electroenceph. Clinical Neurophysiology* 10 (1958):297.

Drucker, P.F. "The New Philosophy Comes to Life." *Harper's Magazine,* August, 1957.

Eccles, J.D., Krnjević, K. "Potential changes recorded inside primary afferent fibers with the spinal cord." *Journal of Physiology* 149: (1959):250–73.

Eisenberg, L. "Medicine—Molecular, Monetary, or More than Both?" *Science* 274 (1995):331–34.

Emerson, R.W. *Literary Ethics,* 1838. In: Emerson, R.W. Centenary Editon (12 vols., 1903-4).

Emery, E.S., Jr., Monroe, R.T. "Peptic ulcer; Nature and treatment based on a study of 1,435 cases." *Archives of Internal Medicine* 55 (1935):271–92.

Engel, B.T., Blecker, E.R. "Application of operant conditioning techniques to the control of the cardiac arrhythmias." In: *Cardiovascular Psychophysiology*, edited by P.A. Obrist, 456–76, Chicago: Aldine, 1974.

Engel, G.L. "How much longer must medicine's science be bound by a seventeenth century world view?" In: White, K.L. *The Task of Medicine.* Menlo Park, CA: Henry J. Kaiser Family Foundation, 1988, p 121.

Engel, F.L., Fredericks, J. *Proceedings Society of Experimental Biology and Medicine* 94 (1957):593.

Ershler, W.B., Sun, W.H., Binkley, N. "The role of interleukin-6 in certain age-related diseases." *Drugs and Aging* 5 (1994):358–65.

Ewing, J.A., Haizlip, T.M. "A controlled study of the habit forming propensities of meprobamate." *American Journal of Psychiatry* 114 (1958):835.

Feldman, P.E. "The personal element in psychiatric research." *American Journal of Psychiatry* 113 (1956):52–54.

Fernel, J.: In: *Man on His Nature.* Sir Charles Sherrington, London: 1951.

Finland, M., Collins, H.S., Wells, E.B. "Aureomycin in the treatment of primary atypical pneumonia." *New England Journal of Medicine* 240 (1949):241–46.

Finney, J.M.T. *A Surgeon's Life.* New York: G.P. Putnam & Sons, 1940.

Fischer, H.K., Dlin, B.M. "The dynamics of placebo therapy: A clinical study." *American Journal of Medical Science* 232 (1956):504–12.

Flavell, G. "Reversal of Pulmonary Hypertrophic Osteoarthropathy by Vagotomy." *Lancet* 1 (1956):260.

Forssman, W. "Die Sondierung des rechten Herzens." *Klin. Wchnschr.* 8 (1929):2085.

Freedman, D.X., Fenichel, G. *A.M.A. Archives of Neurology & Psychiatry* 79 (1958):164.

Friedman, M., Rosenmann, R. "Association of specific overt behavior pattern with blood and cardiovascular findings." *Journal American Medical Association* 169 (1959):1286.

Frost, R. "Mending Wall." In: *Oxford Book of American Verse*. F.O. Matthieson (ed.). p. 547, 1950.

Gall, F.J. *Philosophische medizinische Untersuchungen über Kunst und Natur im gesunden und kranken Zustand des Menschen*. Leipzig, 1800.

Gantt, W.H. "Effect of Person." *Conditional Reflex* 1 (1966):18–34.

Gantt, W.H. "Analysis of the Effect of Person." *Conditional Reflex* (April–June, 1972): 67–73.

Garrison, F.H. *An Introduction to the History of Medicine*. Philadelphia, PA: W.B. Saunders Co., 1929, p. 505.

Gassendi, P. "Syntagma philosophicum (1658)." Cited in Fellows, O.E., and Torrey, N.L. *The Age of Enlightenment: An Anthology of Eighteenth-Century French Literature*, second edition, New York: Appleton-Century-Crofts, 1971, p. 6.

Gibbon, E. *The Decline and Fall of the Roman Empire*. 8 vols. William Pickering: London: Tolboys & Wheeler, Oxford, 1827.

Gliedman, L.H., Gantt, W.H., Teitelbaum, H.A. "Some implications of conditional reflex studies for placebo research." *American Journal of Psychiatry* 113 (1957):1103–07.

Gliedman, L.H., Nash, E.H., Jr., Imber, S.D., Stone, A.R., and Frank J.D. "Reduction of symptoms of pharmacologically inert substances by short-term psychotherapy." *Archives of Neurology and Psychiatry*, 79 (1958):345–51.

Gold, H. and Greiner, T.: "A Method for the Evaluation of the Effect of Drugs on the Cardiac Pain of Angina of Effort. *Journal of Pharmacology and Experimental Therapeutics*, 98(1950), p. 10.

Gooch, G.P. *Frederick the Great*. New York: Dorset Press, 1990.

Gordon, O.L. and Chernya, Y.M. "Physiology of the gastric secretion in man; studies on patients with gastric fistula and artificial esophagus." *Klin. Med.* 18 (1940):63–71.

Gorgas, W.C. *Sanitation in Panama*. New York: D. Appleton Co., 1918, p. 204.

Grace, W.J., Wolf, S., Wolff, H.G. *The Human Colon*. New York: Paul B. Hoeber, Inc., 1951.

Grace, S.J., Graham, D.T. *Psychosomatic Medicine* 14 (1952):243.

Graham, D.T., Wolf, S. "The Pathogenesis of Urticaria. Experimental Study of Life Situations, Emotions, and Cutaneous Vascular Reactions." *Journal American Medical Association* 143 (1950):1396.

Graham, D.T., Stern, J.A., Winskur, G. *Psychosomatic Medicine* 20 (1958):427.

Grant, M.P. *Microbiology and Human Progress*. New York: Rinehart & Co., 1953, p. 638.

Gravenstein, J.S. "Das Leermittel (Placebo) in der klinischen Pharmakologie." *Arzneim-Forsch.* 6 (1956):621–23.

Gravenstein, J.S., Smith, G.M., Sphire, R.D., Isaacs, J.P. Beecher, H.K. "Dihydrocodeine. Further development in measurement of analgesic power and appraisal of psychologie side effects of analgesic agents." *New England Journal of Medicine* 254 (1956):877–85.

Gray, C.M., Freeman, W.J., Skinner, J.E. "Chemical dependencies of learning in the rabbit olfactory bulb: Acquisition of the transient spatial pattern change depends on norepinephrine." *Behavioral Neuroscience* 100 (1986):585–96.

Gregg, A. "The golden gate of medicine." *Annals of Internal Medicine* 30 (1949):810–22.

Groover, M.E. *Transactions College of Physicians of Philadelphia* 24 (1957):105.

Gunn, C.G., Friedman, M., Byers, S.O. "Effect of chronic hypothalamic stimulation upon cholesterol induced atherosclerosis in rabbit." *Journal Clinical Investigation* 39 (1960):1963–72.

Gunn, C.G. Hampton, J.W. "CNS Influence on Plasma Levels of Factor VIII Activity." *American Journal of Physiology* 212 (1968):124–30.

Guyton, A.C. *American Journal of Physiology* 154 (1948):45.

Haffner, S.M., Valdez, R.A., Myukkanen, L., Stern, M.P., Katz, M.S. "Decreased testosterone and dehydroepiandrosterone sulfate concentrations are associated with increased insulin and gluocse concentrations in nondiabetic men. *Metabolism* 43 (1995):599–603.

Haggard, H.W. *Devils, Drugs and Doctors.* New York: Harper & Bros., 1929, p. 364.

Haight, T.H. "Erythromycin therapy of respiratory infections. I. Controlled studies on the comparative efficacy of erythromycin and penicillin in scarlet fever." *Journal of Laboratory and Clinical Medicine* 43 (1954):15–30.

Haight, T.H. Unpublished material.

Halberg, F. *Cold Spring Harbor Symposia on Quantitative Biology* 25 (1960):289.

Haldane, J.B.S., Priestley, J.F. *Respiration.* London: Oxford University Press, 1935.

Halliday, J.L. *Psychosocial Medicine: A Study of the Sick Society.* W.W. Norton Co., New York, 1948.

Hammersten, J.F., Cathey, C.W., Redmont, R. Wolf, S. *Journal Clinical Investigation* 36 (1957): 899 (abstract).

Hammersten, J.F., Cathey, C., Redmont, R., Jones, H., Adsett, C.A., Schottstaedt, W.W., Wolf, S. "The relation of life stress to the concentration of serum lipids in patients with coronary artery disease." *American Journal of Medical Science* 244 (1962):421.

Hammon, W. McD., Coriell, L.L., Stokes, J., Jr. "Plan of Controlled Field Tests and Results of 1951 Pilot Study in Utah." *Journal American Medical Association* 150 (1952):739.

Hampton, J.W., Cunningham, G.R., Bird, R.M. "The pattern of inheritance of defective fibrinase (Factor XIII)." *Journal of Laboratory and Clinical Medicine,* 1966.

Hanzlik, P.J.: "Jan Evangelista Purkyne (Purkinje) on Disturbances of Vision by Digitalis, 100 Years Ago." *Journal American Medical Association* 84 (1925):2024.

Hardy, J.D., Wolff, H.G., Goodell, H. *Pain Sensations and Reactions.* Baltimore, MD: Williams & Wilkins Co., 1952.

Harris, G.W., Woods, J.W. In: *Regulation and Mode of Action of Thyroid Hormones,* G.E.W. Wolstenholme and E.C.P. Millar (eds.) p. 3, Boston: Little Brown & Co, 1957.

Hebert, P.R., Rich-Edwards, J.W., Mason, J.E., Ridker, P.M., Buring, J.E., Hennekens, C.H. "Weight and risk of future myocardial infarction." *Abstracts from 64th Scientific Session. American Heart Association* II (1991):35.

Henle, W. "Studies on Agent of Infectious Hepatitis." *Journal of Experimental Medicine* 92 (1950):271.

Hernandez-Peon, R., Sherrer, H., Jouvet, M. "Modifications of electrical activity in cochlear nucleus during attention in unanesthetized cats." *Science* 123 (1956):331.

Hetzel, B.S. "Thyroid Secretion in Health and Disease." *Australian Annals of Medicine* 13 (1964):80.

Heymans, C. *Perspectives in Biology and Medicine* 3 (1960):409.

Hinkle, L.E., Jr., Conger, G.B., Wolf, S. "Studies on Diabetes Mellitus: The relation of stressful life situations to the concentrations of ketone bodies in the blood of diabetic and non-diabetic humans." *Journal Clinical Investigation* 29 (1950):754.

Hinkle, L.E., Jr., Evans, F., Wolf, S. "Studies in Diabetes Mellitus IV: Life History of Three Persons with Relatively Mild, Stable Diabetes, and Relation to Significant Experiences in their Lives to the Onset and Course of Disease." *Psychosomatic Medicine* 13 (1951):184.

Hippocrates. *Works of Hippocrates. Medical Classics,* vol. 3, Baltimore, MD: Williams & Wilkins, 1938.

Hiro, Y., Tasaka, S. "Die Roteln sind Viruskrankleiten." *Monatschr. Kinderh.* 76 (1938):328.

Hoff, E.C., Greene, C.W. "Cardiovascular reactions induced by electrical stimulation of the cerebral cortex." *American Journal Physiology* 117 (1936):411.

Hoff, E.C., Kell, J.F., Hastings, N., Shales, D.M., Gray, E.H. *Journal of Neurophysiology* 14 (1951): 317.

Hoffman, G.W., Kion, T.A., Grant, M.D. "An idiotypic network model of AIDS immunopathogenesis." *Proceedings National Academy of Science* 88 (1991):3060–64.

Hofling, C.K. "The place of placebos in medical practice." *General Practice*, Kansas City, MO: 11:(1955):103–07.

Holling, H.E., Brodey, R.S., Boland, H.C. "Pulmonary Osteoarthropathy." *Transactions of Association of American Physicians* 73 (1960):305.

Holmes, R.H., Goodell, H., Wolf, S., Wolff, H.G. *The Nose.* Springfield, IL: Charles C. Thomas, 1950.

Holmes, T.H., Hawkins, N.G., Bowerman, C.E., Clark, E.R. Joffe, J.R. "Psychosocial and Psychophysiologic Studies of Tuberculosis." *Psychosomatic Medicine* 19 (1957):134.

Holmes, T.H., Rahe, R.H. "The Social Readjustment Rating Scale." *Journal of Psychosomatic Research* 11 (1967):213–18.

Houssay, B.A., Rietti, C.T., Ashkar, E., et al. "Fatty metabolism and ketogenesis after liver denervation or bilateral thoracolumbar sympathectomy in pancreatectomized dogs." *Diabetes* 16 (1967):259–63.

Huang, M.H., Ebey, J., Wolf, S. "Manipulating the QT Interval of the ECG by Cognitive Effort." *Pavlovian Journal of Biological Sciences* 24 (1989)102–08.

Hubel, D.H., Wiesel, T.N. "Receptive fields of single neurons in the cat's striate cortex." *Journal of Physiology* 148 (1959):574–91.

Hubel, D.H., Wiesel, T.N. "Shape of arrangements of columns in cat's striate cortex." *Journal of Physiology* 165 (1963):559–68.

Huxley, T.H. *Our Knowledge of the Causes of the Phenomena of Organic Nature.* London: Macmillan, 1863.

Hyrtl, J. *Lehrbuch der Anatomie des Menschen mit Rücksich auf physiologische Begründung und praktische Anwendung.* Prague: Ehrlich, 1846.

Imai, H., Taylor, C.B., Werthessen, N.T. "Angiotoxicity and arteriosclerosis due to contaminants of USP grade cholesterol." *Archives of Pathology and Laboratory Medicine* 100 (1976):565–72.

Imai, H. "Report of workshop on study and review of angiotoxic and carcinogenic sterols in processed food." *Research Office and Office of Naval Research* 1977.

Ivy, A.C. "The history and ethics of the use of human beings in medical experiments." *Science* 108 (1948):1.

Jefferson, G. "Man as an Experimental Animal." *Lancet* 1 (1955):59.

Jellinek, E.M. "Clinical Tests on Comparative Effectiveness of Analgesic Drugs." *Biometrics* 2 (1946):87.

Jonsen, A.R. "Humanities are the hormones." *Perspectives in Biology and Medicine* 33 (1989):133–42.

Jordan, S.M., Kiefer, E.D. "Factors influencing prognosis in the medical treatment of duodenal ulcer." *American Journal of Surgery* 15 (1932):472–82.

Kandel, E.R. *The Cellular Bases of Behavior.* San Francisco, CA: Freeman, 1976.

Kelly, H.A. *Walter Reed and Yellow Fever.* Baltimore, MD: Medical Standard Book Co., 1906.

Keys, A., Brozek, J., Henschel, A., Mickelsen, O., Taylor, H.L. *The Biology of Human Starvation,* vol. 1. Minneapolis: University of Minnesota Press, 1950.

Kion, T.A., Hoffman, G.W. "Anti-HIV and anti-anti-MHC antibodies in alloimmune and autoimmune mice." *Science* (1991): 1138–45.

Kneeland, Y., Jr., Rose, H.M., Gibson, C.D. "Aureomycin in the treatment of primary atypical pneumonia." *American Journal of Medicine* 6 (1949):41–50.

Krause, A.K. "Tuberculosis and Public Health." *American Review of Tuberculosis* 18 (1928):271.

Laennec, R. *De L'Auscultation Médiate, ou Traité du Diagnostic des Maladies des Poumons et du coeur, Flordé Principlement sur a Nouveau Moyen d'Exploration.* Paris, 1834.

Lahey, F.H. "The treatment of gastric and duodenal ulcer." *Journal American Medical Association* 95 (1930):313–16.

Lasagna, L., von Felsinger, J.M. "Volunteer Subjects in Research." *Science* 120 (1954):359.

Lasagna, L., Mosteller, F., von Felsinger, J.M., Beecher, H.K. "A study of the placebo response." *American Journal of Medicine* 16 (1954): 770–79.

Lasagna, L. "The controlled clinical trial: Theory and practice." *Journal of Chronic Diseases* 1 (1955):353–67.

Lasagna, L., Laties, V.G., Dohan, J.L. "Further studies on the 'pharmacology' of placebo administration." *Journal of Clinical Investigation* 37 (1958):533–37.

Leape, L.L. "Error in Medicine." *Journal American Medical Association* 272 (1994):1851–57.

Leslie, A. "Ethics and practice of placebo therapy." *American Journal of Medicine* 16 (1954):854–62.

Leuwenhoek, A. van. In: *Source Book of Medical History,* edited by L. Clendening, Toronto: General Publishing Co., 1960, p. 218.

Lewis, Sir Thomas. *Pain.* New York: Macmillan Co., 1942.

Liddle, G.W. "Unexpected cause of Cushing's Syndrome: Carcinomas that secrete ACTH." *Transactions American Clinical and Climatological Association* 74 (1962).

Lilly, J.C. *The Deep Self: The Tank Method of Physical Isolation.* New York: Simon & Schuster, 1977.

Linfors, E.W., Neelon, F.A. "The case for bedside rounds." *New England Journal of Medicine* 303 (1980):1230–33.

Ling, G., Gerard, R.W. "Normal membrane potential of frog sartorius fibers." *Journal of Cell Composition and Physiology* 34 (1949):383–96.

Loosli, C.G. "Medical education and training in research." *Journal of Laboratory and Clinical Medicine* 47 (1956):3.

Lorenz, K. *Evolution and Modification of Behavior.* Chicago: University of Chicago Press, 1965.

Lucretius. *De Natura Rerum* (The Nature of Things), Cyril Bailey (trans.). Cambridge, MA: Loeb Classical Library, 1947.

Lynch, J. *The Broken Heart.* New York: Basic Books, 1977.

Lynch, J. Paskeiwitz, D.A., Gimbel, K.S., Thomas, S. "Psychological aspects of cardiac arrhythmias." *American Heart Journal* 93 (1977):645–57.

Lynch, J. *Living Together: Dying Alone.* New York: Basic Books, 1977.

Macht, D.I. "The History of Intravenous and Subcutaneous Administration of Drugs." *Journal American Medical Association* 66 (1916):856.

MacLean, P.D., Flanigan, S., Flynn, J.P., Kim, C., Stevens, J.R. *Yale Journal Biological Medicine* 28 (1955):380.

Maddox, J. "Research turned upside down." *Nature* (1991) 353:297.

Magendie, F. In: *Behavioral Science in Clinical Medicine,* S. Wolf and H. Goodell (eds.), 1976, pp. 6–7, Springfield, IL: Charles, C. Thomas.

Malpighi, M. "Duae Epitstolae de Pulmonibas." Florence, 1661. Quoted in M. Foster, *Lectures on the History of Physiology.* London: Cambridge University Press, 1901.

Manning, G.W., Hall, G.E., Banting, F.G. *Canadian Medical Association Journal* 37 (1937): 314.

Marey, E.J. "Decomposition des phases d'un Mouvement au Moyen l'images photographiques successives receuillies sur une bande de papier sensible qui se deroule." *Compte Rendus Academie Science* 103 (1886):509.

Martini, P. "Die unwisentliche Versuchsanordnung und der sogenannte doppelt Blindversuch." *Dutch Medicine Wschr.* 82 (1957):597–602.

Masserman, J. Personal communication, 1954.

McCulloch, W. "Introductory Discussion." In: *Cybernetics,* Foerster, H. von (ed.). New York: Josiah Macy Jr. Foundation, 1950.

McDougal, J.B. *Tuberculosis—A Global Study in Social Pathology.* Baltimore, MD: Williams and Wilkins, 1949.

Meiklejohn, G., Shragg, R.I. "Aureomycin in primary atypical pneumonia. A controlled evaluation." *Journal American Medical Association* 140 (1949):391–96.

Minot, G.R., Murphy, W.P. "A Diet Rich in Liver in the Treatment of Pernicious Anemia: A Study of 105 Cases." *Journal American Medical Association* 89 (1927):759.

Miracle drugs. Current editorial comment. *New York State Journal of Medicine* 53 (1953):1740.

Mirick, G.S., Leftwich, C.I., Henle, G. "Apparent Failure of Material from Chick Embryos Inoculated with Hepatitis (IH) Virus to Immunize Against Unadapted Virus." *Transactions Association of American Physicians* 67 (1954):293.

Mitchinson, M.J., Ball, R.Y., Carpenter, K.L.H., Parums, D.V. "Macrophages and ceroid in atherosclerosis." In: *Hyperlipidemia and Atherosclerosis*, K.E. Suckling and P.H.E. Groot (eds.). London: Academic Press, 1988.

Mock, D.C., Jr. "Variability of Diuretic Response as Influenced by State of Organism: Note on Law of Initial Values." *American Journal of Medical Science* 238 (August 1959):193–201.

Modell, W. "The relief of symptoms." In: Bockus, *Gastroentenology*. Philadelphia, PA: W.B. Saunders, 1955, ch. 4.

Modell, W., Houde, R.W. "Factors influencing clinical evaluation of drugs. With special reference to the double-blind technique." *Journal American Medical Association* 167 (1958):2190–99.

Moorman, L.J. "Tuberculosis on the Navaho Reservation." *American Review of Tuberculosis* 61 (1950):586.

Moorman, L.J. 1954, personal communication.

Morales, A.J., Nolan, J.J., Nelson, J.C., Yen, S.S. "Effects of replacement dose of dehydroepiandrosterone in men and women of advancing age." *Journal of Clinical Endocrinology Metabolism* 78 (1994):1360–67.

Morris, J.N. "Coronary Heart Disease and Physical Activity of Work." *Lancet* 265 (1953):1053.

Moser, R. "Alarums and lamentations." *Transactions of American Clinical & Climatological Association* 91 (1979):43.

Mountcastle, V.B., Bloom, F.E., Geiger, S.R. (eds.) *Handbook of Physiology: The Nervous System III*. Baltimore, MD: Williams & Wilkins, 1984.

Muller, S. "An interview with Steven Muller." *U.S. News and World Report*, November 10, 1980, p. 57.

Nash, O. *Humor from Harper's*, John Fischer and Lucy Donaldson (eds.). New York: Harper and Brothers, 1961.

Negoescu, R.M., Csiki, I.E., Pafnote, M. "Stabilizing the rate: a straight cortical repercussion of the heart." *IEEE-IMBS* 11 (1989):147–52.

Nestler, J.E., Clore, J.N., Blackard, W.G. "Dehydroepiandrosterone: the 'missing link' between hyperinsulinemia and atherosclerosis? *FASEB Journal* 6 (1992):3073–75.

Olshaker, B., Ross, S., Recinos, A. Jr., Twible, E. "Aureomycin in the treatment of pneumonia in infants and children." *New England Journal of Medicine* 241 (1949):287–95.

Ornstein, R. (ed.). *The Healing Brain*. New York: Guilford, 1990.

Osler, W. "On the need for a radical reform in our methods of teaching senior students." *Medical News* 82 (1903):49–50.

Osler, W. *The Old Humanities and the New Sciences.* Boston: Houghton Mifflin, 1920.

Osler, W. Quoted in R. Dubos, *Mirage of Health,* p. 120, New York: Harper & Bros. 1959.

Palinski, W. "Low density lipoprotein undergoes oxidative modification in vivo." *Proceedings National Academy of Science* 86 (1989):1372–76.

Palmer, R.W. "The hypotensive action of Rauwolfia serpentina and reserpine: A double hidden placebo study of ambulatory patients with hypertension." *American Practitioner* 6 (1955):1323–27.

Pandya, D.N., Yeterian, E.H. In: *Cerebral Cortex of Man,* vol. 4, Peters, A., Jones, E.G. (eds.). New York: Plenum, 1985.

Paracelsus "De Moto Pharmacandi." In: *Paracelsus,* F. Hartman, John W. Lowell (trans.). Reprinted 1963 by Health Research, Mohlumne Hills, CA.

Parkes, C.M. "Bereavement." *British Medical Journal* 3:(1967):232.

Parkinson, C.N. "Haste and Waste in Science." *Think* (February, 1960): 24–27.

Parson, W. "Questions and Reflections." *The Pharos* (1995):34.

Parsonnet, J., Friedman, G.D., Vandersteein, D.P., Chang, Y., Vogelman, J.H., Orentreich, N., Sibley, R.K. "Helicobacter pylori infection and the risk of gastric carcinoma." *New England Journal of Medicine* 325 (1991):1127–31.

Parsons, R.P. *Trail to Light: A Biography of Joseph Goldberger.* Indianapolis, IN: Bobbs-Merrill Co., 1943, pp. 296–313.

Pavlov, I. *Conditioned Reflexes: An Investigation of the Physiological Activity of the Cerebral Cortex,* G.V. Anrep (trans.). New York: Oxford, 1927.

Peabody, F. *Doctor and Patient: Papers on the Relationship of Physicians to Men and Institutions.* New York: Macmillan, 1930.

Pepper, O.H.P. "A note on placebo." *American Journal of Pharmacology* 117 (1945):409–12.

Pette, D., Düsterhöft, S. "Altered gene expression in fast-twitch muscle induced by chronic low-frequency stimulation." *American Journal of Physiology* 262 (1992):R333-R338.

Pickering, G. In: *Frontiers in Hypertension Research,* J. Laragh, F. Buler (eds.). 1981, p. 38.

Pickering, G.W. "Concepts of medical education abroad as they relate to cardiovascular teaching—and—modern concepts in the teaching of cardiopulmonary function and disease." *Fifth Conference on Cardiovascular Training Grant Program Directors,* Williamsburg, VA, 1958, p. 11.

Pidoux, H. Quoted in *Mirage of Health* by R. Dubos, New York: Harper, 1959.

Pierpaoli, W., Regelson, W. *The Aging Clock.* New York: The New York Academy of Science, vol. 719, 1994.

Pinel, P.Y. *The Clinical Training of Doctors: An Essay of 1793,* D. Weiner (ed. and trans). Baltimore, MD: The Johns Hopkins University Press, 1908.

Pinel, P *Nosographie philosophique, 1800, ou la méthode de l'analyse appliquée à la médecine,* second edition. Paris: J.A. Brosson, 1803.

Pinsker, H.M., Kupfermann,I., Castellucci, V., Kandel, D. *Science* 167 (1970):1740.

Pinsker, H.M., Willis, W.D. *Information Processing in the Nervous System.* New York: Raven Press, 1980.

Platt, J.R. "Strong Inference." *Science* 146 (1964):347–54.

Plimpton, C.H. "The Hidden Strength Within." Inaugural address, Amherst College, October 30, 1960.

Poeggeler, B., Reiter, R., Tan, D.X., Chen, L.D., Manchester, L.C. "Melatonin, hydroxyl radical-medicated oxidative damage, and aging: a hypothesis." *Journal Pineal Research* 14 (1993):151–68.

Pound, R.: "The Professions in the Society Today." Lecture to the Massachusetts Medical Society. *New England Journal of Medicine* 241 (1949):351–57.

Portugal, F.H., Cohen, J.S. *A Century of DNA: A History of the Discovery of the Structure and Function of the Genetic Substance.* Cambridge, MA: MIT Press, 1977, p. 141.

Rahe, R.H., McKean, J., Arthur, R.J. "A longitudinal study of life changes and illness patterns." *Journal of Psychosomatic Research* 10 (1967):355.

Rapport, S., Wright, H. (eds.). *Great Adventures in Medicine.* New York: Dial Press, p. 271.

Rauws, E.A.J., Tytgat, G.N.J. "Cure of duodenal ulcer associated with eradication of Helicobacter pylori." *Lancet* 335 (1990):1233–35.

Reiter, R. Personal communication.

Rees, W.D., Lutkins, S.G. "Mortality of Bereavement." *British Medical Journal* 4 (1967):13.

Reid, D.D. "The design of clinical experiments." *Lancet* 2 (1954):1293–96.

Reifenstein, G.H. "Rheumatic-like lesions found in unselected autopsies." *Proceedings American Federation for Clinical Research* 4 (1948):2.

Reiter, R., Tan, D,-X., Poegeler, B., Chen, L.-D, Menendez-Pelaez, A. "Melatonin, free radicals and cancer initiation." In: *Advances in Pineal Research,* Maestroni, G.J.M., Conti, A., Reiter, R. (eds.). London: John Libbey, 1994.

Richet, C. "La résistance des canards à l'asphyxie." *Comptes Rendus de las Société de Biologie* 1 (1894):244–45.

Richet, C. "Défense de l'organisme contre les traumatismes." *Revue Scientifique* 53 (1894):259.

Rinzler, S.H., Travell, J., Bakst, H., Benjamin, Z.H., Rosenthal, R., Rosenfeld, S. Hirsch, B. "Effect of heparin in effort angina." *American Journal of Medicine* 14 (1953):438–47.

Rothstein, W.G. *American Medical Schools and the Practice of Medicine: A History.* New York: Oxford University Press, 1987.

Rowe, W.P. "Protective effect of pre-irradiation on lymphocytic choriomeningitis infection in mice." *Proceedings Society of Experimental Biology and Medicine* 92 (1956):194.

Rushmer, R.F., Smith, O.A. "Cardiac Control." *Physiological Reviews* 39 (1959):41–68.

Russek, J.E., Zohman, G. *American Journal of Medical Science* 235 (1958): 266.

Russell, G.F., Hill, J.I. "Odor differences between anantiomeric isomers." *Science* 172 (1971):1943–44.

Russian Scientific Translation Program. "The central nervous system and human behavior." *National Institutes of Health,* 1959.

Sacks, O. "Neurology and the Soul." *The New York Review of Books,* November 22, 1990:44–50.

Scheibel, A.B., Wechsler, A.B. (eds.). *Neurobiology of Higher Cognitive Function.* New York: Guilford, 1990.

Schelenz, C. "Ut aliquid fieri videatur." *Münich Med. Wschr.* 100 (1958):944–45.

Scherf, D., Boyd, L.J. *Clinical Electrocardiography.* Philadelphia, PA: Lippincott, 1946.

Schonbach, E.B., Bryer, M.S. "Treatment of primary atypical nonbacterial pneumonia with aureomycin." *Journal American Medical Association* 139 (1949):275–80.

Schottstaedt, W.W., Pinsky, R.H., Mackler, D. "Sociologic, psychologic and metabolic observations on patients in the community of a metabolic ward." *American Journal of Medicine* 25 (1958):248.

Schottstaedt, W.W., Grace, W.J., Wolff, H.G. *Journal Psychosomatic Research* 1 (1956):203.

Schottstaedt, W.W., Pinsky, R.H., Mackler, D. "Prestige and social interaction on a metabolic ward." *Psychosomatic Medicine* 21 (1959):131.

Schottstaedt, W.W., Jackman, N.R., McPhail, C.S. "Prestige and social interaction on a metabolic ward; the relation of problems of status to chemical balance." *Journal of Psychosomatic Research* 7 (1963):83–95.

Schneider, R.A., Costiloe, J.P., Wolf, S. "Arterial pressures recorded in hospital during ordinary daily activities. Contrasting in subjects with and without ischemic heart disease." *Journal of Chronic Diseases* 23 (1971):647–57.

Schroeder, H.A. "Why not control hypertension with drugs?" *Clinical Research Proceedings* 3 (1955):1–5.

Science News Letter, February 23, 1957, p. 127.

Sechenov, I. *Reflexes of the Brain*, (Moscow, 1873). Reprinted by Idz-Vo Academy of Medicine, USSR, 1952.

Sechenov, I.M. *Selected Works*. Moscow: All Union Institute for Experimental Medicine, 1935.

Seifter, J., Baeder, D., Zarafonetic, C., Kalas, J. In: *Hormones and atherosclerosis*, G. Pincus (ed.). New York: Academic Press, 1959.

Sendrail, M., "L'Homme à L'Hôspital." *Concours Mèdecine* 76 (1954):4193.

Seyle, H. *The physiology and pathology of exposure to stress*. Montreal: Acta, Inc., 1950.

Shapiro, A.P., Grollman, A. "A critical evaluation of the hypotensive action of hydralazine, hexamethonium, tetraethylammonium and dibenzyline salts in human and experimental hypertension." *Circulation* 8 (1953):188–98.

Sheldon, W.H. *Presidential Address, Southern Society for Clinical Research*. January, 1956.

Sheldon, M.B. Personal communication.

Sherrington, C.S. *The Endeavor of Jean Fernel*. Cambridge: Cambridge University Press, 1946.

Shimkin, M.G. "The Problem of Experimentation on Human Beings I. The Researcher's Point of View." *Science* 117 (1953):205.

Sigerist, H.E. *Man and Medicine*, Margaret Galt Boise (trans.). New York: William V. Norton, 1932.

Simmons, L.W., Wolff, H.G. *Social Science in Medicine*. New York: Russell Sage Foundation, 1954.

Skinner, J.E., Martin, J.L., Landisman, C.E., Mommer, M.M., Fulton, K., Mitra, M., Burton, W.D., Saltzberg, B. "Chaotic attractors in a model of neocortex: dimensionalities of olfactory bulb surface potentials are spatially uniform and event-related." In: *Brain Dynamics Progress and Perspectives* (1990):119–34.

Skinner, J.E., Goldberger, A.L., Mayer-Kress, G., Ideker, R.E. "Chaos in the heart: Implications for clinical cardiology." *Biotechnology* 8 (1990):1018–24.

Skinner, J.E. "Neurocardiology: Brain Mechanisms Underlying Fatal Cardiac Arrhythmias." *Neurology Clinician* 11 (1993):325–51.

Smith, W.O., Duvall, M.K., Joel, W., Honska, W.L., Wolf, S. "Further studies on experimentally induced atrophic gastritis in dogs." *Transactions Association of American Physicians* 73 (1960):348–55.

Smithwick, R.H., Castleman, B. "Some Observations on Renal Vascular Disease in Hypertensive Patients Based on Biopsy Material Obtained at Operation." In: Bell, E.T. (ed.) *Hypertension*. Minneapolis: University of Minnesota Press, 1951.

Snow, C.P. *The Two Cultures and the Scientific Revolution.* New York: Cambridge University Press, 1961.

Spencer, S.M. *Wonders of Modern Medicine.* New York: McGraw-Hill Book Co., 1953.

Speransky, U.D. *A Basis for the Theory of Medicine.* New York: International Publishers, 1943.

Sprinkle, R.H., *Profession of Conscience.* Princeton, NJ: Princeton University Press, 1994.

Stamler, J., Pick, R., Katz, L.M. "Experiences in Assessing Estrogenic Antiatherogenesis in the Chick, the Rabbit and Man." *Annals of New York Academy of Medicine* 64 (1956):463.

Staum, M.S. *Cabanis: Enlightenment and Medical Physiology in the French Revolution.* Princeton, NJ: Princeton University Press, 1980.

Steel, K., Gertman, P.M., Crescenzi, C. et al. "Iatrogenic illness on a general medical service at a university hospital." *New England Journal of Medicine* 304 (1981):638–42.

Stein, E. *The Electrocardiogram.* Philadelphia, PA: W.B. Saunders, 1976.

Steinberg, D. "Beyond cholesterol. Modifications of low-density lipoprotein that increase its atherogenicity." *New England Journal of Medicine* 320 (1989):915–24.

Steiner, J. In: *Wein M. Wchnschr.,* 25 (1875):305.

Stokes, J., Jr. "Carrier State in Viral Hepatitis." *Journal American Medical Association* 154 (1954):1059.

Straub, L.R., Ripley, H.S., Wolf, S. "Disturbances in Bladder Function in Association with Varying Life Situations and Emotional Stress." *Journal American Medical Association* 141 (1949):1139–43.

Stroebel, C.F., Glueck, B.C. "Biofeedback treatment in medicine and psychiatry: An ultimate placebo?" *Semin Psychiatry* 5 (1953):379–92.

Strohman, R.C. "Linear genetics and non-linear adaptations in cells: Limits of genetic predictability in biology and medicine. *Integrative Physiological and Behavioral Sciences* 30 (1995).

Strong, R.P. *Philippine Journal of Science* 1 (1906):512.

Sutherland, A.M. "Psychological impact of cancer surgery." Washington, DC: *Public Health Report,* p. 1139, 1952.

Sutherland, E.W. "On the biological role of cyclic AMP." *Journal American Medical Association* 214 (1970):1281–88.

Tang, J., Wolf, S. "Proteolytic Enzymes of the Gastric Juice Organic Constituents in Human Gastric Juice." *Gastroenterology* (1968):186–94.

Taylor, K.B. "Autoimmune Phenomena in Pernicious Anaemia: Gastric Antibodies." *British Medical Journal* 2 (1962):1347–52.

Teilhard de Chardin, P. *The Phenomenon of Man.* London: Collins, 1955.

Thomas, D. *The Doctors and the Devils.* New York: James Laughlin, 1953, p. 131.

Time, July 30, 1945, p. 46.

Tibbetts, R.W., Hawkings, J.R. "The placebo response." *Journal of Mental Science* 102 (1956):60–66.

Tosteson, D.C. "New pathways in general medical education." *New England Journal of Medicine* 332 (1990):234–38.

Traut, E.F., Passarelli, E.W. "Placebos in the treatment of rheumatoid arthritis and other rheumatic conditions." 16 (1957):18–22.

Trudeau, E.L. *An Autobiography.* New York: Doubleday, Page, and Co., 1916.

Tuteur, W. "The 'double blind' method: Its pitfalls and fallacies." *American Journal of Psychiatry* 114 (1958):921–25.

Tyler, D.B. "The effect of amphetamine sulfate and some barbiturates on the fatigue produced by prolonged wakefulness." *American Journal of Physiology* 150 (1947):253–62.

Utkin, I.A. *Theoretical and practical questions of experimental medicine and biology in monkeys.* New York: Pergamon Press, 1958.

Vaihinger, H. *The Physiology of "As If,"* C.K. Ogden (trans.). London: Rutledge, 1949, p. 12.

Valbona, C., Cardus, D., Spencer, W.A., Hoff, H.E. "Patterns of sinus arrhythmia in patients with lesions of the central nervous system." *Journal of Laboratory and Clincial Medicine* 16 (1965):379–89.

Virchow, R. *Disease, Life and Man.* Stanford, CA: Stanford University Press, 1958.

Voltaire. *Candide and Other Writings.* New York: The Modern Library, 1956.

Walker, S.H. "Ineffectiveness of aureomycin in primary atypical pneumonia. A controlled study of 212 cases." *American Journal of Medicine* 15 (1953):593–602.

Walter, W.G. *The Living Brain.* New York: W.W. Norton & Co. 1953, p. 275.

Weiner H., Hofer, M.A., Stunkard, A.J. (eds.). *Brain, Behavior, and Bodily Disease, Research Publications.* Association for Research in Nervous and Mental Diseases, vol. 59. New York: Raven Press, 1981.

Wenckebach, K.F., Winterberg, H. *Die Unregelmassige Hertztatigkert.* Leipzig: Engelmann, 1927.

Wiersma, E.D. "Der Einfluss von Bewustesinszustünden auf den Puls und auf die." *Atmung. Zeit. Ges. Neurological Psychology* 19 (1913):1–24.

Wernicke, E. Footnote in Kolle and Wassermann's *Handbuch der Pathogenen Mikoorganismen,* 1913.

Whitcomb, W.H. "Erythropoietic Factor in Hypoxic Patients with Emphysema without Secondary Polycythemia." *Archives Internal Medicine* 103 (1959): 871.

Wiener, N. *Cybernetics, or Control and Communication in the Animal and the Machine.* New York: John Wiley, 1948.

Windholz, G. "Schilder and Pavlov's theory of higher nervous activity: A critique and an apologia." *Integrative Physiological and Behavioral Science* 26 (3) (1991):248–58.

Witts, J. "Research and the Patient." *Lancet* 1 (1955):1115.

Wolbach, S.B., Todd, J.L., Palfrey, F.W. *The Etiology and Pathology of Typhus.* Being the main report of the Typhus Research Commission of the League of Red Cross Societies to Poland. Cambridge: Harvard University Press, 1922.

Wolf, S. "The relation of gastric function to nausea in man." *Journal of Clinical Investigation* 22 (1943):877–82.

Wolf, S., Wolff, H.G. *Human Gastric Function: An Experimental Study of a Man and His Stomach.* New York: Oxford University Press, 1943; second edition, 1947.

Wolf, S. "Observations on the occurrence of nausea among combat soldiers." *Gastroenterology* 8 (1947):15–18.

Wolf, S., Pfeiffer, J.B., Ripley, H.S., Winter, O., Wolff, H.G. "Hypertension as a reaction pattern to stress: Summary of experimetnal data on variations in blood pressure and renal blood flow." *Annals of Internal Medicine* 29 (1948):1056–76.

Wolf, S., Almy, T. "Experimental Observations on Cardiospasm in Man." *Gastroenterology* 13 (1949):401.

Wolf, S. "Summary of evidence relating life situation and emotional response to peptic ulcer." *Annals Internal Medicine* 31 (1949):637.

Wolf, S. "Effects of suggestion and conditioning on the action of chemical agents in human subjects—The pharmacology of placebos." *Journal of Clinical Investigation* 29 (1950):100–09.

Wolf, S., Holmes, T.H., Treuting, T., Goodell, H., Wolff, H.G. "An experimental approach to psychosomatic phenomena in rhinitis and asthma." *Journal of Allergy* 21 (1950):1–11.

Wolf, S. "Mechanisms underlying some epigastric symptoms." *Journal American Geriatric Society* 1 (1953):813–20.

Wolf, S., Pinsky, R.H. "Effects of placebo administration and occurrence of toxic reactions." *Journal American Medical Association* 155 (1954):339–41.

Wolf, S. "The evaluation of therapy in disease." *Transactions American Clinical and Climatological Association* 66 (1955):61.

Wolf, S., Cardon, P.S. Jr., Shepard, E.M., Wolff, H.G. *Life Stress and Bodily Disease.* Baltimore, MD: Williams & Wilkins, 1955.

Wolf, S. "Lest one good custom." editorial, *Clinical Research Proceedings* 4 (1956):166.

Wolf, S., Doering, C.R., Clark, M.L., Hagans, J.A. "Chance distribution and the placebo reactor." *Journal of Laboratory and Clinical Medicine* 49:837, 1957.

Wolf, S. *The Evaluation of Therapeutic Agents.* Washington, DC: American Psychiatric Mental Hospital Service, 1957.

Wolf, S. "The evaluation of therapeutic agents with special reference to the tranquilizing drugs." *Monogoraph Series no. 2, APA Mental Hospital Service,* January, 1957.

Wolf, S. "Placebos: The effect of pharmacological agents on the nervous system." *Association for Research in Nervous and Mental Diseases,* 37 (1959):147–61.

Wolf, S. "The pharmacology of placebos." *Pharmacological Reviews* 11 (1959):689–704.

Wolf, S. "Disease as a way of life: Neural integration in systemic pathology." *Perspectives in Biology and Medicine* 4 (1961):288–305.

Wolf, S. "Changes in serum lipids in relation to emotional stress during control of diet and exercise." *Circulation* 26 (1962):379.

Wolf, S. "A new view of disease." *Journal of American Medical Association* 184 (1963):129.

Wolf, S. *The Stomach.* Oxford: Oxford University Press, 1965.

Wolf, S. "The bradycardia of the dive reflex. A possible mechanism of sudden death." *Conditional Reflex* 2 (1967):88–95.

Wolf, S. "Psychosocial forces in myocardial infarction and sudden death." *Circulation* (Suppl.) 4 (1969):39–40; 74–83.

Wolf, S. "Emotions and the autonomic nervous system." *Archives of Internal Medicine* 126 (1970):1024–30.

Wolf, S., Grace, K.L., Bruhn, J.G., Stout, C. "Roseto revisited: Further data on the incidence of myocardial infarction in Roseto and neighboring Pennsylvania communities." *Transactions of American Clinical and Climatological Association* 85 (1974):100–08.

Wolf, S., Goodell, H. *Behavioral Science in Clinical Medicine.* Springfield, IL: Charles C.Thomas, 1975.

Wolf, S., Wolf, T.D. "A preliminary study in medical anthropology in Brunei, Borneo." *Pavlovian Journal* 13 (1978):42–54.

Wolf, S. "The Role of the Brain in Bodily Disease: Insights from the Convergence of Neurobiology and Behavioral Science" In: *Proceedings Association of Research in Nervous and Mental Diseases,* New York: Raven Press, 1980.

Wolf, S. and Berle, B.B. (eds.). *The Technological Imperative in Medicine.* New York: Plenum Press, 1981.

Wolf, S. "The stomach's link to the brain." *Federation Proceedings* 44 (1985):2889–93.

Wolf, S., Bruhn, J.G. *The Power of Clan.* New Brunswick, NJ: Transaction Publishers, 1993.

Wolf, S. "Oscillatory functions affecting outcome of coronary heart disease." *Integrative Physiological and Behavioral Science* 30 (1995):118–26.

Wolff, H.G. "Tuberculosis Mortality and Industrialization." *American Review of Tuberculosis* 42 (1940):1.

Wolff, H.G., Hardy, J.D., Goodell, H. "Studies on pain: Measurement of the effect of morphone, codeine, and other opiates on the pain threshold and an analysis of their relation to the pain experience." *Journal of Clinical Investigation* 19 (1940) 659.

Wolff, H.G., Goodell, H. "The relation of attitude and suggestion to the perception of and reaction to pain." *Proceedings of the American Research of Nervous and Mental Disorders* 23 (1943):434.

Wolff, H.G., DuBois, E.F., Gold, H. "Cornell Conferences on Therapy: Use of placebos in therapy." *New York State Journal of Medicine* 46 (1946):1718–27.

Wolff, H.G., Wolf, S., Hare, C.C. *Life Stress and Bodily Disease. Proceedings of the Association for Research in Nervous and Mental Diseases.* Baltimore, MD: Williams & Wilkins, 1949.

Wolff, H.G. *Stress and Disease*, Springfield, IL: Charles C. Thomas, 1952.

Wolff, H.G. *Headache and Other Pain.* New York: Oxford University Press, 1962.

Woodward, T.E. "Chloromycetin and aureomycin: Therapeutic results." *Annals of Internal Medicine* 31 (1949):53–82.

Wright, A.D. "Clinical Research." *Transactions Medical Society of London* 72 (1956):1.

Glossary

Action potential. Electrical charge developed in a cell during activity.

Alveolar septa. Walls of the pulmonary air sacs where oxygen is absorbed and exchanged for carbon dioxide.

Anaphylaxis. A severe and potentially fatal allergic reaction.

Aplasia. A marine crustacean widely used to study neurophysiology.

Atrophic gastritis. Chronic atrophy of the mucous membrane of the stomach.

Axon. Extension of a neuron by which impulses travel.

Baroreceptors. Transmitter of force from one cell to another.

Chemoreceptors. Capable of transferring a chemical effect to another cell.

Cochlear nucleus. The central receptive site of auditory impulses.

Cytokines. Energy transmitting agents that are released by cells of the immune system.

Dendrites. Branching extensions of neurons that constitute its receptive surface.

Dendritic development. Lengthening and branching of dendrites that enhance the field of intercommunication in the brain.

Enzymes. Proteins capable of implementing or producing a chemical reaction.

Epigenetic. Occurring after the initial expression of genes.

Fourth ventricle. The area at the base of the brain from which the nerves for many visceral regulatory mechanisms emerge.

Gastrocnemius. The lateral muscle of the calf.

Gastric resection. Surgical removal of part of the stomach.

Gastroenterostomy. Surgical attachment of the stomach to the small intestine.

Hippocampus. A brain site concerned with learning and memory.

Homeostasis. Approximate stability in the regulatory bodily mechanisms.

Hyperemesis gravidarum. Vomiting of pregnancy.

Hypertrophic pulmonary osteoarthropathy. Bony excrescences on the fingers and long bones associated with chest diseases.

Hypothalamus. An area on the base of the brain that receives messages from the cortex and mediates bodily regulatory functions.

Ligand. A molecule that donates electrons to form bonds with metallic ions.

Locus ceruleus. A site near the base of the brain that contains noradrenergic neurons.

Metabolism. The production of energy to maintain a living organism.

Mitral Stenosis. Narrowing of the valve opening between the left auricle and ventricle of the heart.

Myocytes. Muscle cells.

Neural transmitter. One of a number of peptide and other molecules that transmit pulses from one cell to another.

Neurokinin. A peptide released from a blood plasma protein that can stimulate pain nerves.

Neuronal plexus. A network of interactive neurons.

Neurons. Conducting cells of the nervous system.

Noise. Random disturbance in an electric circuit.

Olfactory cortex. The site where smell sensations are processed.

Optic cortex. The site where visual sensations are processed.

Osmoreceptors. Capable of transferring a change in the concentration of particles in a solution.

Placebo. A substance without biological action used in the treatment of a patient's symptoms or to balance a drug in a therapeutic experiment.

Presystolic rumble. a rough sound that precedes the first heart sound. It is characteristic of heart damage caused by rheumatic fever.

Receptors. A cell surface that is capable of receiving from one and attaching to another cell.

Redox equilibrium. Acid-base equilibrium.

Refractory period of the heart muscle. A short interval before the next beat during which the heart cannot be stimulated.

Reticular activating system. A brain site concerned with consciousness and the processing of sensations.

Rheumatic nodules. Rounded subcutaneous lumps seen in rheumatic fever or rheumatoid arthritis.

R waves. Electrocardiographic feature that reflects the depolarization of the ventricles.

Sinus arrhythmia. Variability in the timing of the heart beat.

Soleus. The medial muscle of the calf.

Solitary nucleus. A site in the base of the brain where information from visceral afferent nerves is received.

Synaptic transmission. The transfer of an impulse from one neuron to another across a narrow gap via a chemical messenger.

Thalamus. A brain center for sensory impulses that are transferred to the cortex.

Trophic. nourishing.

Tropic. altering.

Vagus nerve. The tenth cranial nerve that participates in the regulation of most of the viscera.

Name Index

Subject Index